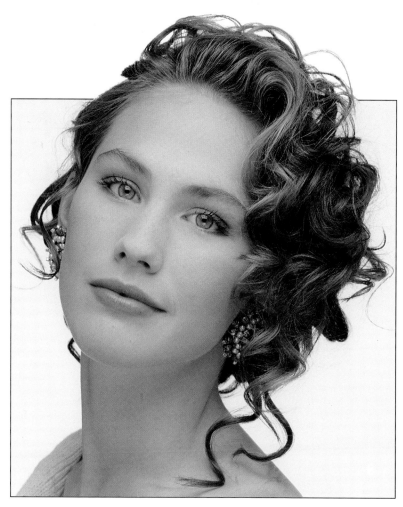

HOME
HAIRSTYLING
MADE EASY

A STEP-BY-STEP GUIDE TO GREAT LOOKING HAIR

HAMLYN

First published in 1992 by Paul Hamlyn Publishing Limited, part of Reed International Books Limited, Michelin House, 81 Fulham Road, London SW3 6RB

Copyright © GE Fabbri 1992

ISBN 0 600 57561 6 (hardback)
ISBN 0 600 57562 4 (paperback)

A catalogue record for this book is available from the British Library.
....

CONTENTS

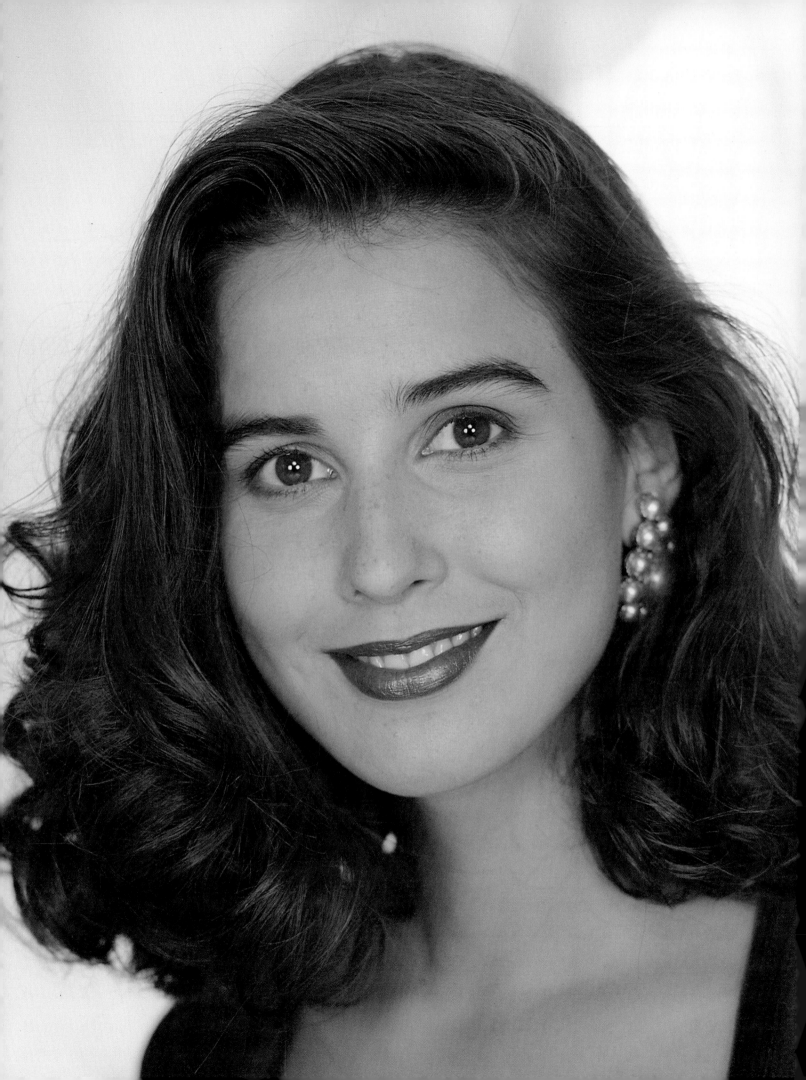

How many times have you wondered how to get your hair looking the way you want it to? **HOME HAIRSTYLING MADE EASY** answers all your styling queries from techniques to great new ideas. Here in one fact-filled, lavishly illustrated book is the information you need to keep your hair, and your man's hair, in tiptop condition.

Our **BASIC HAIRCARE** quiz is designed to help you work out your hair type and the best ways to cope with it. Your face shape can make all the difference to the hairstyle you choose, so compare your face shape with our simple guide and you won't go wrong. You can find information on the right way to wash your hair, step-by-step to conditioning and advice on how to trim your hair and solve problems such as split ends.

A great way to beautiful hair is to know how to use accessories. Follow our advice in **YOUR ESSENTIAL KIT** and find out how best to use YOUR hairstyling accessories.

There's more to drying your hair than you think. Check out the facts on scrunching and other drying methods in **DRYING TECHNIQUES** . Ever puzzle over what to use on your hair? We give you the lowdown in **MOUSSE, GEL, WAX & SPRAY,** what the products are and how to use them.

Finally, ring the changes with your hair without going to the hairdresser. Whatever the length of your hair, in **SIMPLE STYLES** there are suggestions for you to try. Our illustrated, step-by-step instructions make any style easy and you can create a *new you* in a very short time.

HOME HAIRSTYLING MADE EASY answers all your questions, gives you tips and advice and helps you to get the best results with your hair - and it allows you to do it all in your own home!

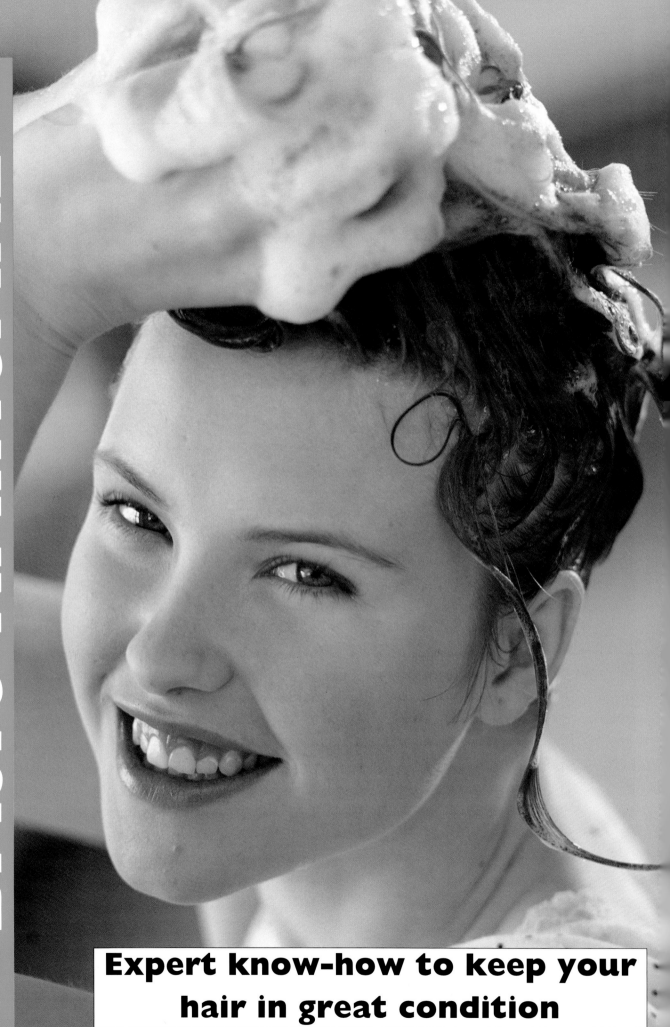

BASIC HAIRCARE

Expert know-how to keep your hair in great condition

KNOW YOUR HAIR

How much do you really know about your hair? You probably think you know if it's dry or greasy, but there's a lot more to learn. And it's worth knowing, because the key to successful styling is knowing what you will, or more importantly won't be able to do with your hair

Read through the questions below and either tick the answer which best describes your locks, or put your hair through a series of simple tests. Then check your score to discover your hair type and how it should be treated so it always looks good.

CAN YOU HANDLE IT?

When you wash your hair and then dry it naturally, what happens to it? Does it:

Hang down without any shape or movement? ☐
Have natural wave or curl? ☐
Look full of life and bouncy? ☐
Look wiry? ☐

When your hair's just been washed and is still wet, pull out a single hair, taking care not to stretch it. Lie the hair on a flat surface, like a mirror, and leave it to dry without touching it. Once dry, has it:

Stayed completely straight? ☐
Curled around slightly? ☐
Twisted like a corkscrew? ☐

Watchpoint

When pulling out a hair, try to hold it as close to your scalp as possible and pull sharply. Don't twist as you pull as this will distort the hair.

Take a smooth roller and when you've washed your hair, wind a few strands around the roller.

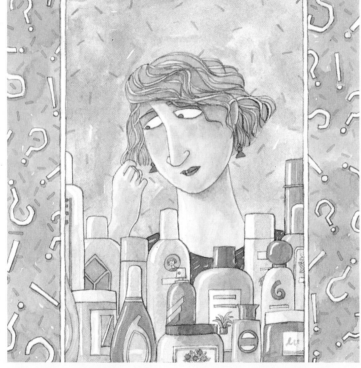

Then leave it to dry naturally. How long does it take for the curl to drop out?

Less than a day ☐
A couple of days ☐
About a week ☐

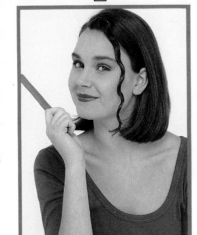

On average, how long would you say you spend getting your hair the way you want it in the morning?

5 minutes or less ☐
10 minutes ☐
15 minutes ☐
20 minutes or more ☐

Does your hair have static? In other words, does it ever lift up and follow the comb as you move it away?

Yes ☐
No ☐

Would you describe your hair as having a mind of its own?

Yes ☐
No ☐

Does your hair stand up a little at the roots?

Yes ☐
No ☐

Can you run your fingers through your hair to freshen up the style?

Yes ☐
No ☐

RESULTS

YOU SCORED MOSTLY ☐
You're lucky! Your hair is easy to handle and tends to do what you tell it. But you've still got to treat it right, because it'll soon become unmanageable if you don't!
- Choose products to suit your hair type: dry, oily, normal, permed or coloured.
- Try different ways of styling your hair – blow-dry, finger-dry, and use tongs.

YOU SCORED MOSTLY ☐
Your hair isn't all that easy to handle so there's no point in attempting the impossible. The trick is to go with what you've got, rather than try to force it into a style it doesn't want to stay in.
- Go for either short or long styles, mid-length is always more difficult to look after.
- Try setting the hair on rollers then blow-drying it as you brush your hair afterwards.
- Buy some gel/mousse/wax and try it out when you next style your hair – it may help you to control it better.

7

GREASE IS THE WORD

Brush your hair back from your face and look at it closely in the mirror. Tick the answer which best describes how it looks:

The whole length of the hair is dull, with no sheen at all. ■

The whole length of the hair seems to be glossy. ■

The roots look shiny but the ends are dull. ☐

With the hair still held back, smooth your fingers along the length, working away from your face. How does it feel?

Slightly springy? ☐

Rough to touch? ■

Smooth and slippy? ■

Wash and dry your hair as usual, but don't use any conditioner or styling products, like mousse or spray. In the evening, split a tissue in half so that it's only one layer thick and gently hold it against your scalp. Can you see any trace of oil left on the tissue:

On the first evening? ■

If not, don't wash your hair and try again. Can you see oil:

On the next evening? ■

On the following morning? ■

On the third evening? ☐

On the fourth morning? ☐

On the fifth evening? ■

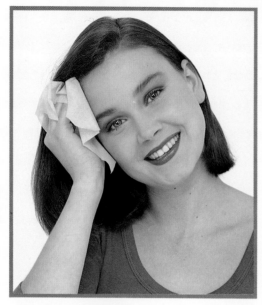

RESULTS

YOU SCORED MOSTLY ■
Your hair probably feels dry and coarse, can be hard to comb and tends to lack lustre and shine.

You're often disappointed because it looks dull, can be flyaway and prone to damage – especially split ends.

● Don't be scared to wash your hair every day, providing you use the right type of shampoo it will not make it any drier – it may even help. Massage will help the natural oils to move down the hairshaft.

● Use a rich, cream shampoo but only give your hair one wash. Condition every time, using a preparation formulated for dry, damaged hair. If your hair's long, comb through to the ends and try to leave the conditioner on for at least a minute. Use an intensive conditioning treatment at least once a month, and try to leave it on for 30 minutes.

● Leave your hair to dry naturally whenever possible. Treat very gently when wet and only ever use a wide-toothed comb. Always use a styling mousse (or a heat styling lotion) with added conditioners before blow-drying, and keep your dryer on a low setting.

● Take vitamin B or brewer's yeast tablets every day to help encourage a healthy shine (vets give it to dogs for dull coats!)

YOU SCORED MOSTLY ■
Your hair tends to look flat, lank and doesn't hold a style very well. This is often due to upset hormones – oily hair is usually worse during a person's teens and early twenties, as well as before periods.

● Wash your hair every day – oily hair tends to pick up more dirt than other types and can smell, but don't massage too much as it increases the oils. Special shampoos are available which dry up the oils. Don't use hot water as it's thought to encourage the sebaceous glands to produce more oil.

● You probably don't need a conditioner after every wash, unless your hair is long. If it is, use a conditioner from the mid-

---

A QUESTION OF CONDITION

Pull a single hair from your head, hold it up to the light and examine it closely. Are there any flimsy bits peeling away about half way up the hair?

Yes ■

No ■

Does the end of the hair look blunt and the same thickness as the rest (as opposed to getting thinner and tapering off)?

Yes ■

No ■

How often do you use heated styling appliances, like tongs, crimpers or heated rollers?

Every day ■

Every couple of days ■

About once a week ■

For the odd special occasion ■

How often do you have a perm, highlights or permanent colour?

Never? ■

Very occasionally? ■

Often – more than three times a year? ■

Do you use conditioner:

Every single time that you wash your hair? ■

Every now and then? ■

Never? ■

Put a ruler on the table. When your hair's freshly washed and still wet, pull out a single hair and hold it firmly at one end of the ruler. Gently stretch the

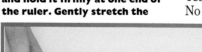
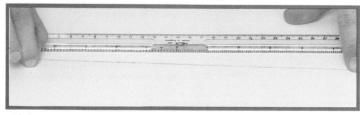

hair by pulling the other end. Does it:

Stretch about one third or more of its original length? ■

Break before it reaches one third? ■

Do you use an intensive, or special conditioner:

Once a week? ■

About once a month? ■

Only ever once or twice? ■

Never? ■

When you study a strand of your hair, do the roots look shiny but the ends of your hair look dull?

Yes ■

No ■

RESULTS

YOU SCORED MOSTLY ■
Your hair isn't in brilliant condition. It's probably difficult to comb when it's wet, and has a tendency to tangle. It feels coarse, and can look slightly fuzzy and matt – it won't have much shine.

● Use a conditioner every time you wash your hair, to help put back the shine and make it more manageable. Choose the one that best suits your hair type: frequent-use lotions are best for oily hair: normal hair creams for dry, colour-treated or permed hair.

● Use an intensive (oil or wax based) conditioning treatment twice a month.

● Spray-on conditioners that aren't washed out are great for dry ends and give a boost to curls and perms in particular.

length to the ends only, and avoid putting any on your scalp.
• Don't overload your hair with lots of dirt-attracting styling products. Choose layered styles, rather than one-length, because they're easier to add body to and won't look so limp. Avoid fringes and styles which leave hair around your face.
• Use spirit-based conditioning lotions to dry up the oils.

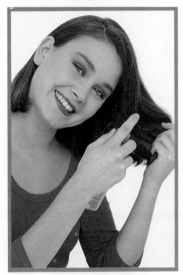

YOU SCORED MOSTLY ☐
You're lucky, you've got the easiest type of hair to deal with and it suits most styles. Your

Take care not to use too much if you've got very fine hair, and unless your hair is very thick, don't use them very close to the scalp.
• Always use a heat styling lotion or styling mousse before blow-drying to help protect your hair from the heat of the dryer. Don't use heated stylers too often and check your brushes and combs regularly for rough edges that may split and tear your hair.
• If you've got long hair that's dry at the ends, use one of the dry ends creams. These have an extra thick formulation, which you just put onto the bottom couple of inches of hair to condition it.
• Avoid perming or chemical colouring treatments: they won't help your hair's condition at all. Go for vegetable colours, especially shades of red, and

hair looks shiny, without having particularly oily roots or over-dry ends.
Wash your hair as often as it needs it. Use a frequent-wash shampoo – you'll only need to wash your hair once.
Use a conditioner as needed, but if you've got long hair be sure to use it at least on the ends – they'll be a bit drier than the rest. And if your hair ever feels tangled or is hard to comb when wet, you must use a conditioner.
Try a spray-on conditioner that you don't wash out after applying. A light formulation won't overload your hair.
Treat yourself to an occasional deep conditioning treatment to maintain the texture and shine.
Normal hair is usually quite strong, so it takes colouring and perming well. But if you want it to stay normal, don't subject it to more than three chemical treatments a year. Opt for vegetable-based colours not chemically based and always test before next chemical/vegetable treatment.
Don't use heated styling products too often.

natural rinses to make your hair look shiny.

YOU SCORED MOSTLY ☐
Your hair's in good shape. It looks healthy and shiny, and will take colour or perms well. But don't be complacent, it'll soon go out of condition if you don't keep up the good work:
• Use conditioners regularly – the right one for your hair type when you wash, and an intensive conditioning treatment once a month.
• Trim your hair regularly – this will help keep the style, and make sure you never suffer from split ends.
• Don't overdo the permanent colour or perms – if you do use chemical treatments on your hair, make sure it's less than three times a year.
• Check that the shampoo you're using isn't too harsh.

IS IT THICK OR THIN?

Pull out a long hair and tightly wind it along an orange stick for about 2 mm. Then count how many times it'll wrap around.
Up to 15? ☐
16-30? ☐
31 and over? ☐

Pull out another hair. Hold it between your finger and thumb, leaving about 2-3 cm/¾-1¼ in sticking out. Does it:
Bend over the side without any natural support? ☐
Stand up straight? ☐
Support itself for about 1 cm/ ⅓ in before bending? ☐

Sit in front of a mirror with the light, preferably daylight, behind you. Part your hair down the middle and take hold of a few hairs – about 1 cm/⅓ in square. Lift them straight up by holding the ends of the hair. Does the hair look:

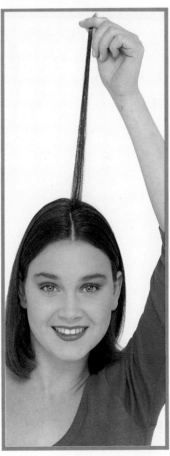

So tightly packed together that you cannot see through it? ☐
Quite transparent and easy to see through? ☐

Difficult to see through. It parted easily, but no light seems to be shining through your hair? ☐

RESULTS

YOU SCORED MOSTLY ☐
Lots of people envy someone with very thick hair, but you know how annoying it can be. The trick is not to fight your hair's natural movement – make the most of its natural texture and accept that it'll never look really smooth and sleek. Although your hair's likely to be quite resistant to colours and perms, which means the processing might take longer, the results are always worth it because they tend to last longer on thick hair than on any other hair types.
• Stick to short styles. If you like your hair long, stick to one-length styles, or ones with long layers (short layers tend to stick out).
• Go for techniques like scrunching and fingerwaving.
• Coarse hair needs regular conditioning to prevent it looking frizzy. Pick the right products to suit your hair type.

YOU SCORED MOSTLY ☐
Your hair tends to look limp very quickly, so regular trims are a must to keep it in shape. Choose a style that needs minimum attention – a short crop or one-length bob are both ideal. Your hair will look thicker if it swings free of your shoulders, so unless you really love long hair, keep it at jaw level or above.
• Consider highlights, they will help to add texture and body to your hair. All-over lighteners aren't a good idea because fine hair tends to be delicate and susceptible to damage.
• Avoid all-over curly perms. If your hair's at all fragile they may encourage it to break or go frizzy. But a body or root perm will work well.
• Use a heat styling lotion or mousse before you style – thin hair is particularly prone to flyaway ends.

A good hairstyle is all about disguising your bad points and playing up your good. You probably feel quite familiar with the face that stares back at you every morning, but try asking a handful of friends what shape they think it is and you're likely to get a handful of answers. The best way to find out is to test its shape yourself. Your face should fall into one of five basic categories: oval, round, square, heart-shaped or long. If you've got an oval face aren't you the lucky one because any style should suit you. If you haven't, then you'll need to spend a little time finding a hairstyle that makes the most of your face.

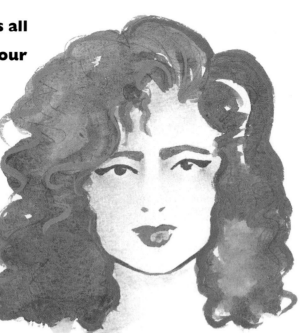

Square-shaped faces *are complemented by wavy hair which frames them.*

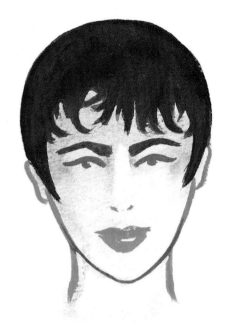

Heart-shaped faces *look best with shorter hairstyles which emphasise the smallness of the chin.*

FACE VALUES

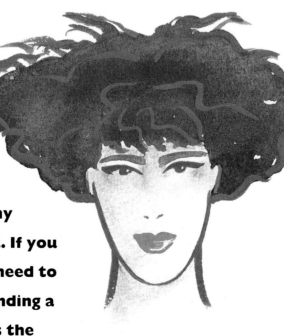

Long-shaped faces *call for short, wide hairstyles to balance their length.*

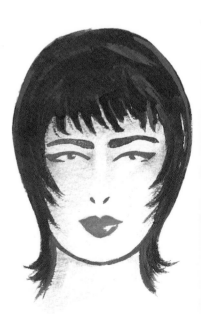

Round-shaped faces *need simple hairstyles to frame them and give the impression that they are smaller.*

TRACE YOUR FACE

Probably the easiest and most effective way to find your face shape is to scrape your hair from your face (use a hairband or scarf if necessary) and look closely in a well-lit mirror. Then using a lipstick or a soft eye pencil, draw a line on the mirror around the outline of your reflection. When you stand away from the mirror you'll be able to see which category your face shape falls into.

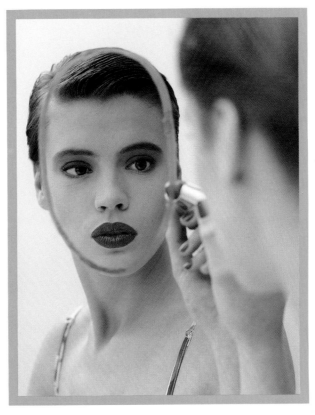

FACE ACHES

Learn how to disguise your own particular problem area.

- Big ears: choose a style that gives volume at the sides.
- Big nose: opt for a layered fringe and softly layered styles to draw attention away from it.
- High forehead: never style hair away from face. Instead opt for a full or layered fringe.
- Low forehead: avoid emphasising your forehead with an off-the-face style. Go for a full fringe instead.
- Double chin – there's no need to cover up with polo necks and scarves – choose a style that falls onto your face and that isn't cut above chin level.
- Eyes close together: try to avoid styles with a heavy fringe. Instead go for an upswept look. that's styled away from the face.
- Small face: don't overwhelm delicate features. Wear your hair off your face and style it to give height on top and plenty of volume at the sides.

FACE SHAPE	CHOOSE	AVOID
Heart – wide cheekbones and a broad forehead tapering down into a small, often quite pointed, chin.	Wavy or straight short bobs. Short and spiky styles. Unstructured, wispy fringes will divert attention away from wide foreheads.	Any style with a middle parting or a very short fringe. They will make your forehead look even broader.
Square – doesn't mean that you've got a face like Frankenstein's, but that you've got a fairly broad jawline that is often squarish in shape and roughly the same width as your cheekbones.	Wavy or curly styles. Styles that are dried falling onto the face. Side partings. Fringes combed away from the face – these are the perfect complement to this face shape.	Geometric shapes. Long bobs with heavy fringes. Very short cuts. Severe styles where hair is scraped off the face and centre partings.
Long – generally with a long chin or a high forehead.	Styles with fringes to shorten the effect of a long face. Chin-length scrunch-dried or curly bobs that'll balance a long face.	Long, straight, one-length styles. Styles pulled severely off the face. These will only draw attention to your chin and forehead.
Round – the cheeks are the widest part of the face. Having a round-shaped face needn't mean you are overweight.	Unfussy styles with height on top. Bobs that are flicked out below jawline. Styles worn on the face. Side partings.	Bubbly perms and ringlets. Swept-back styles. These have the effect of making the face look rounder.

SHAPE UP

The shape of your face is one of the most important considerations when choosing a new hairstyle, but you should also take into account your overall body shape.

- *Traditional English pear-shapes should not go for cropped elfin styles or anything similar. They will only draw attention to the bottom half of your body – making your head look small for your body and your hips even wider.*
- *Big-busted girls should also avoid very cropped styles and go for a full head of hair instead. Unless, or course, you want to draw attention to your chest!*
- *Very petite girls should try to avoid having masses of very curly hair – it'll probably make your head look too big for your little body!*

Illustrations: ANDREA BYRNE

Is your hair dry and frizzy, and looks beyond repair?

Then treat it to a new hi-tech conditioner and

get it super soft and shiny in a flash!

HAIR SAVERS

Modern styling techniques can take their toll on the look and feel of your hair. Even if you make the effort to slap on a generous blob of conditioner after every shampoo, it's not always enough to correct the damage that's been done. Therefore, it's a good idea to switch to one of the hair-saving conditioners which are specially formulated to coat the hair shaft and leave you with hair that's beautifully manageable and silky smooth.

Follow our guide to the best products around and choose the one that's most suitable for your type of hair.

HOT OIL

This treatment revitalises dry, brittle hair, protects it against further damage, and is the ideal solution for fragile, permed or coloured hair.

Since the oil treatment is used before shampooing, it won't leave a greasy residue. Everyone will benefit from a once a month treatment, but if your hair is badly damaged, you should use it as often as once a week.

▶ Put an unopened tube of hot oil treatment into a cup of hot tap water for a minute or two to warm up.

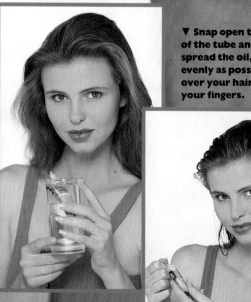

▼ Snap open the top of the tube and spread the oil, as evenly as possible, over your hair using your fingers.

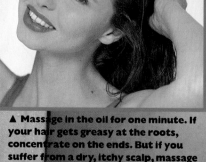

▲ Massage in the oil for one minute. If your hair gets greasy at the roots, concentrate on the ends. But if you suffer from a dry, itchy scalp, massage the oil in with the pads of your fingers. Shampoo as usual.

12

CONDITIONING MOUSSE

Look out for the latest conditioning mousses, which are suitable for all hair types. They tend to be fairly cheap to use since you can accurately control how much you need and where you want the mousse to go. The advantage of conditioning mousse is that it doesn't have to be rinsed out and many contain a built-in sunscreen to help prevent your hair drying out. The foam is light and can be used both to condition your hair and control it if it's flyaway.

▶ Wash your hair and towel-dry it. Make sure you rinse your hair properly so there's no shampoo left in it.

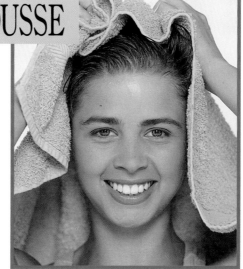

▼ Shake the can of mousse and squirt a blob into your palm – use an egg-sized blob on short to mid-length hair; an orange- to grapefruit-sized blob on longer styles. If you're just conditioning the ends of your hair, go for an egg-sized blob.

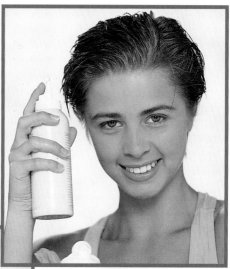

COMB OUT

The whole business of shampooing and massaging in conditioners can leave some nasty tangles in your hair. Rinsing won't remove these knots and by the time you come to styling your hair, you could damage it by having to tug at the tangles. That's why it's a good idea to comb your hair while the conditioner is still in it. This not only makes it more manageable and easy to style afterwards but it also distributes the conditioner, so it coats each strand evenly. Remember, however, to use a wide-toothed comb. Hair is not very elastic when it's wet and may snap, instead of springing back, if it's stretched by a fine-toothed comb.

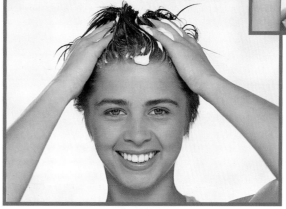

▲ Smooth the mousse between your hands and massage it through your hair from the roots to the ends. Then comb it through with a wide-toothed comb. It'll form a protective coating on your hair and encourage gloss and shine. ▶

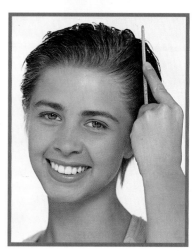

CREAM CONDITIONER

These are great pick-me-ups for dry hair. But their rich, waxy consistency may leave fine hair lank and lifeless. They can be used as often as you need – even after every shampoo – until your hair improves.

Be generous with the conditioner and use plenty to cover your hair.

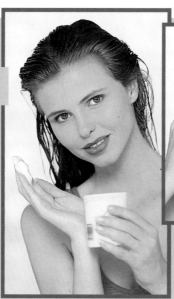

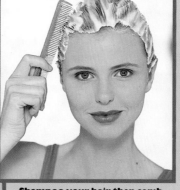

Shampoo your hair then comb through a cupful of conditioner. Leave on for three to five minutes then rinse out.

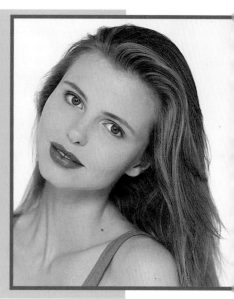

SUPER SERUM

Serums are the latest products on the market designed to deal with dry, split ends. The soft, liquid gel dissolves into an oil conditioner that is massaged into the ends of the hair only. It's claimed that the serums form a delicate film around dry, brittle ends, allowing the active ingredients to moisturise, strengthen and even rebuild the hair tips! The serum doesn't need to be rinsed out and is non-sticky and non-greasy. It leaves hair shiny and easy to style. It's best used twice weekly.

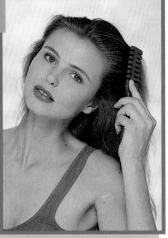

▲ **Brush your hair through to remove any tangles.**

◄ **The serum can be put on either dry hair or slightly damp, towel-dried hair.**

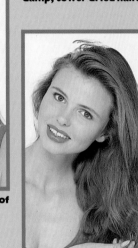

▶ **Squeeze out a pea-sized blob of serum and run it between your fingertips until it turns into a liquid gel. Then massage it into the ends of your hair.**

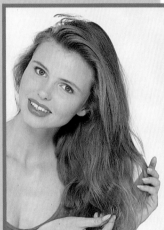

◄ **If your hair is already dry, simply style it into place. But if it's only towel-dried, blow-dry and style your hair as usual.**

If your hair is curly use a serum designed for it, they tame frizz and make it manageable.

Many other intensive conditioners are made from natural ingredients, such as henna, wax, seaweed or mud. These contain proteins and minerals which are claimed to strengthen the hair shaft. They need only be used occasionally.

THE GREEN ALTERNATIVE

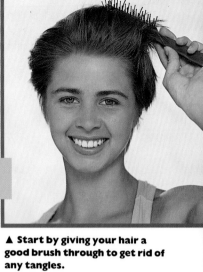

▲ **Start by giving your hair a good brush through to get rid of any tangles.**

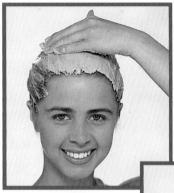

◄ **Scoop out a generous handful of the conditioner and massage it into your scalp, as well as your hair, since the herbal ingredients can treat scalp problems too.**

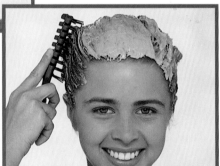

▶ **As the conditioner has to be left on on for 30 minutes, or more if possible, it's best to gather up your hair on the top of your head. The thick consistency of the conditioner will keep it plastered in place. But if your hair is very long, try tucking it under a plastic shower cap.**

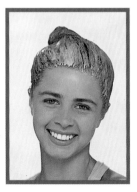

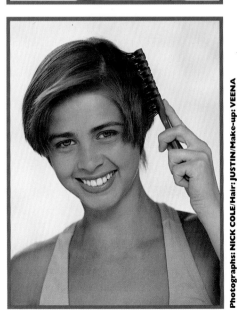

▶ **When the time's up, rinse out the conditioner, then shampoo your hair as usual. If your hair is very dry follow with a light conditioner which can be rinsed out.**

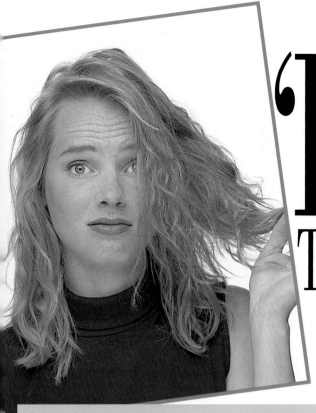

'HELP I CAN'T DO A THING WITH MY HAIR'

Split ends? Dry hair? Growing out a perm?

Don't despair – try our instant and long-term

solutions to make your hair a shining example

SPLIT ENDS

'I've not taken proper care of my hair and now I've got really bad split ends. What should I do about them?'

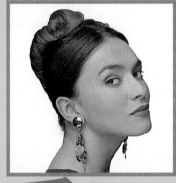

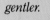

Long hair is often lighter at the ends if you've spent time in the sun. An upswept style creates a flattering contrast between light ends and dark roots.

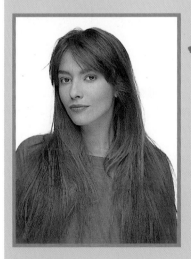

SHORT TERM

Keep them out of sight in a bun or a French pleat where all the ends are covered. Avoid voluminous, curled styles which can emphasise the bushy appearance of split ends.

LONG TERM

There is only one way to get rid of split ends and that's with a regular trim every six weeks. Avoid creating more splits by learning to blow-dry your hair in sections, with the dryer pointing downwards. This technique

smooths the cuticle so that your hair looks its shiny best and can protect itself from further damage.

Also, don't hold the dryer too close to your hair, since it can cause it to dry out and make the ends split. Let your hair dry naturally as often as possible and when putting it up, don't pull it or twist it too tightly. Never use ordinary elastic bands, covered ones are much gentler.

GROWING OUT COLOUR

'I had my hair coloured two months ago and now it's two-toned. How can I cover up the different shades?'

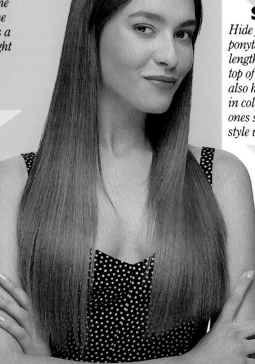

SHORT TERM

Hide your roots! Try a high ponytail or a tousled bun so the length of your hair is piled up on top of your head. Layered looks also help to break up contrasts in colour whereas sleek smooth ones show them off – so choose a style with care.

LONG TERM

If you want to stay the same colour, ask your hairdresser to retouch your roots. To grow the colour out, ask for the ends to be dyed back to your natural shade. A short, layered style breaks up the colour differences.

15

GROWING OUT LAYERS

'I'm trying to grow out my layers, but my hair looks a mess. What can I do about it?'

SHORT TERM

Make the most of your hair's volume so that you have a full look without sharp, neat edges which would emphasise the layers. Tip your head forwards and dry your hair so that you create root lift and a tousled effect, or try scrunch-drying to make soft curls. Long fringes can be dried away from your face and secured with a slide or back-combed and worked into the rest of your hair.

LONG TERM

Regular trims are essential to even up the layers and to allow your hairdresser to start shaping your hair, as it grows, into the new style you'll eventually have – it'll stay tidier too. The growing-out period may be slightly longer than if you leave your hair to do it's own thing, but it will look much better.

THIN HAIR

'My hair is very fine and straight, so any style I try flops quickly. It just seems to go flat whatever I do. Please help me!'

SHORT TERM

You can add a certain amount of temporary body to fine hair by working mousse or thickening lotion through your hair before blow-drying it and then finishing with a spritz of firm-hold hairspray. Make the most of smooth, sleek styles or try sweeping your hair into a loose bun, French pleat or high ponytail on top of your head.

LONG TERM

You can't, of course, change the texture of your hair, but a good cut can help. Long layers can create body at the ends of your hair, while short layers can add lift to the roots. If you want curl as well as volume, try a root perm on shorter hair, or a body perm on longer.

OLD PERM

'How can I cope with my frizzy, growing-out perm ends and new 'flat' roots?'

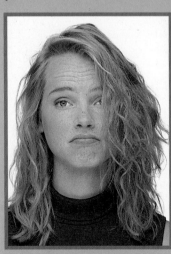

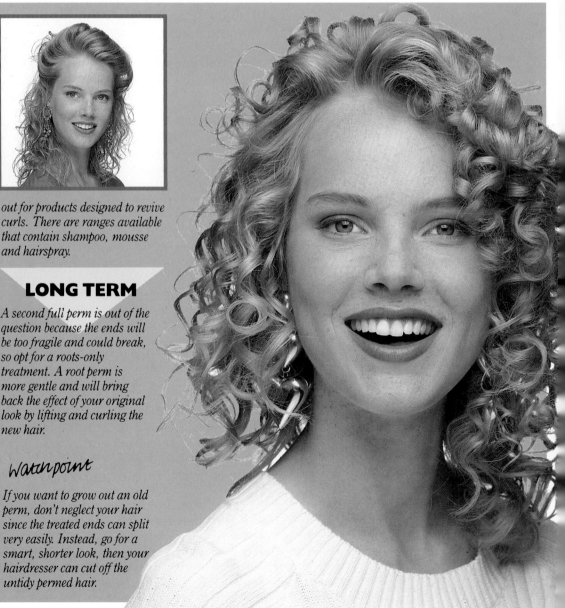

out for products designed to revive curls. There are ranges available that contain shampoo, mousse and hairspray.

LONG TERM

A second full perm is out of the question because the ends will be too fragile and could break, so opt for a roots-only treatment. A root perm is more gentle and will bring back the effect of your original look by lifting and curling the new hair.

SHORT TERM

After washing and conditioning your hair, work in an orange-sized blob of mousse then scrunch-dry the ends to shape and boost the curls for the rest of the day. Add height to straight roots by sweeping your hair up at the front and securing it with a slide. Also, look

Watchpoint

If you want to grow out an old perm, don't neglect your hair since the treated ends can split very easily. Instead, go for a smart, shorter look, then your hairdresser can cut off the untidy permed hair.

OILY HAIR

'My hair is oily and I don't have the time to wash it every day to keep it looking at its best. Any suggestions?'

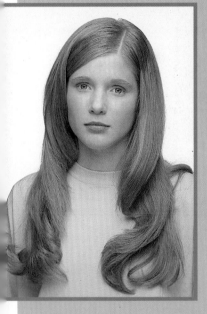

SHORT TERM

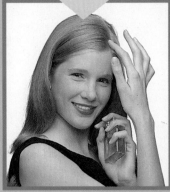

If you are going out straight from the office, try to style your hair as simply as possible, since too much brushing and handling spreads the oil.

Dab a few drops of cologne along your parting or around the hairline where oiliness shows most clearly – the alcohol will dry up some of the oil, and the scent will mask the smoky smells that tend to stick to oily hair. You could also try using a dry shampoo which will absorb some of the oil, but make sure you brush it all out thoroughly.

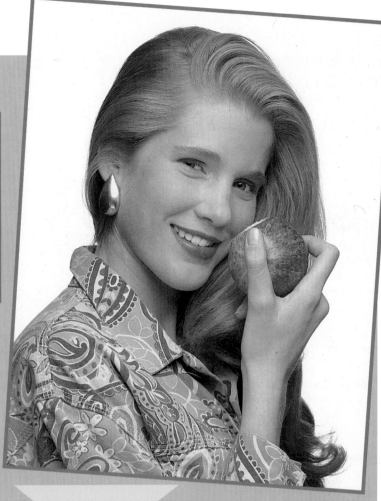

LONG TERM

Oily hair is caused by over-active sebaceous glands which produce the hair's natural lubrication, sebum, and is most common during puberty. The best remedy is to keep yourself really fit so your body can cope with any changes. Try to exercise regularly, have early nights, avoid smoking and drinking, and eat healthily.

THICK HAIR

'I have long, thick hair and even combing it can be a problem, let alone styling or shaping it. Can you help me?'

SHORT TERM

Don't attempt fussy styles, instead take full advantage of your hair's natural volume and go for sweeping looks.

If you fancy an elegant style for evenings, use a little gel to smooth down the roots and then simply plait or twist it up into a bun. Or braid your hair into a thick plait and decorate it with a scrunchie.

LONG TERM

Careful cutting and layering can thin out thick hair. Alternatively, go for a style that depends upon the hair's weight to look good – a blunt-cut bob, a long, tousled look or a graduated cut, for instance. If your hair tends to fall over your face, ask your hairdresser to create a feathered face-framing style for you.

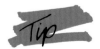

Very thick hair tends not to reflect much light, so brighten it up with a temporary colourant in a rich shade which complements your own hair colour.

DRY HAIR

'My hair is dull and dry. What can I do to get it looking shiny and healthy again?'

SHORT TERM

Make sure you always rinse your hair thoroughly to remove any traces of shampoo. Avoid styling products that dull the surface of your hair – mousse and hairspray can both cause problems, and switch to products that shine as they style – wet-look gel and wax are good to use.

Use a mild, frequent-use shampoo so you don't strip the hair of natural oil and follow with a rich, creamy conditioner.

LONG TERM

If your hair is only dry at the ends it probably just needs trimming and could benefit from using a nourishing conditioner twice weekly. A hormone imbalance at certain times of the month can sometimes cause dryness. So if your hair is dry all over, you should be careful about your diet. Eat lots of fresh fruit and vegetables as well as nuts, pulses and yeast foods which are rich in the healthy hair vitamins B and C. Also, stimulate the circulation by massaging your scalp thoroughly and regularly with your fingertips.

Photographs: PAUL MITCHELL/Hair: JUSTIN/Make-up: KARIN DARNELL/Blue top: DAMART/Orange T-shirt: TOP SHOP/Maroon top: NEXT/Spotted dress: ZOO/Orange wrap top: ZOO Earrings: ACCESSORIZE/White sweater: WAREHOUSE/Earrings: ACCESSORIZE/Green T-shirt: TOP SHOP/Black dress: ZOO/Earrings: ZOO/Earrings: ACCESSORIZE/Jacket: C17/Earrings: ACCESSORIZE

THE RIGHT SHAMPOO FOR THE JOB

It's important that you know your hair type if you want to get the best results possible from your shampoo.

If you have been using styling products that aren't water soluble, like waxes, put the shampoo on your hair before you wet it. By doing this, you will emulsify the oils before you start washing and make any styling products a lot easier to remove.

NORMAL HAIR

This is healthy and manageable. If it's fine, it may have quite a lot of static.

Use a mild shampoo formulated for frequent use and look out for shampoos with added ingredients like grapefruit or lemon which have a slightly astringent quality and will clean and refresh your scalp.

Two-in-one shampoo and conditioners are ideal for normal hair that doesn't need a great deal of conditioning. They can also make normal hair a lot easier to comb through after washing if it's prone to tangles and knots.

DRY HAIR

This hair type tends to look dull, coarse and lack-lustre and if it's long it will probably have split ends. It is often quite unmanageable and prone to static. The scalp may also be dry and flaky. Dry hair needs washing carefully as it is particularly vulnerable to damage. Choose a rich, cream shampoo with conditioning ingredients like jojoba oil. You'll only need a small blob of shampoo – just concentrate on the scalp, not the ends and rinse thoroughly. Remember, just because your shampoo produces lots of lather, this doesn't mean the shampoo is any more effective or richer. Manufacturers often add lathering agents to shampoos because most people think that more lather means cleaner hair.

If your hair is very dry, massage your scalp with warm almond oil before you shampoo – this stimulates blood circulation and acts like a protective coating for the scalp and roots. Then apply a mild shampoo and rinse off as usual.

COMBINATION HAIR

This is a common problem for long hair and means that your hair is oily at the scalp and dry at the ends. Use a mild shampoo that cleans gently, removing oil from the scalp without overdrying the ends. Hair that's prone to oiliness becomes oilier and more limp as the weather warms up so you may have to wash it more in the summer.

If your hair is below shoulder length, never pile it up on top of your head while you're washing or you'll be asking for a mass of tangles.

GREASY HAIR

This is lank, dull and difficult to manage. It clings to the scalp and sometimes smells as it traps sebum, sweat and dirt. The greasies are most common during adolescence when the sebaceous glands are over active and provide too much natural oil (sebum). Unfortunately there is no way of curing over-active sebaceous glands, you'll just have to wash more often. As a temporary measure, stop your scalp and hair smelling by cutting up a lime into slices and rubbing it over your hair and scalp.

If you suffer from dandruff, the specially formulated anti-dandruff shampoos on the market are extremely effective and should clear the problem up in a few weeks. But avoid using anti-dandruff shampoos all the time as they tend to dry out your hair. Use them once a week and alternate with a frequent use shampoo until your scalp is clear. If the problem persists, go and see your doctor.

WASHING ROUTINE

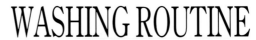

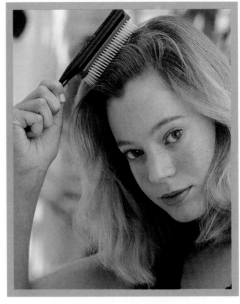

1 **Brush your hair through thoroughly to get rid of tangles and loosen any dead skin cells on your scalp. Soak your hair with warm water using a shower attachment.**

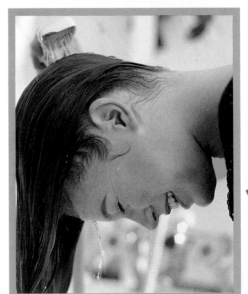

4 **Rinse your hair in warm water, don't stop until the water going down the drain is completely clear.**

Always rinse your hair thoroughly – any residue of shampoo or conditioner will leave it lack lustre and dull.

SPECIAL SHAMPOOS FOR COLOURED HAIR

You can buy shampoos that are made specifically for different coloured hair. They won't actually change the colour of your hair but they should enhance its natural highlights. The henna-based ones designed for red hair tend to produce the most noticeable results.

CHEMICALLY TREATED

If your hair has been bleached, permed, coloured or straightened choose a rich shampoo for treated hair to help keep it in good condition.

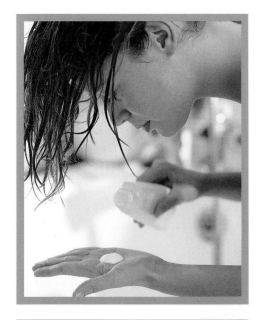

2 Pour a dollop of shampoo that's the size of a big button into one hand then rub your palms together. This ensures the shampoo is evenly distributed instead of going on in one big blob.

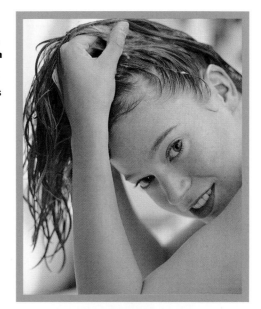

3 Using the pads of your fingers, massage the shampoo into your hair and scalp. Concentrate on your scalp and the hair nearest to it. Don't put shampoo down the length of your hair, there's no need.

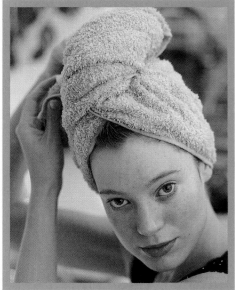

5 When you've rinsed out all the lather, give your hair a final rinse in cold water to encourage a healthy shine. Wrap your hair in a towel, turban style.

Watchpoint

Do not pull or rub the hair during washing as hair is very vulnerable when wet.

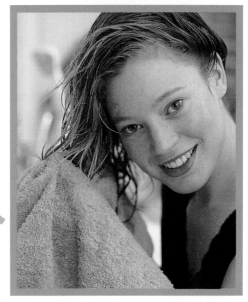

6 Gently blot your hair dry with the towel. Don't rub or you'll end up with tangles and you risk damaging your hair.

Tip

There's no need to shampoo your hair twice unless it's really greasy or dirty.

Tip

If your hair is chemically treated, look out for special conditioning shampoos for permed or colour-treated hair.

GREEN CLEAN

If you are concerned about looking after the environment, choose a biodegradable shampoo that breaks down naturally and doesn't contain any harmful pollutants.

USE OF DRY SHAMPOOS

There really isn't anything to equal thorough shampooing for good looking and fresh-smelling hair. But if you really haven't got time to do this, then try a dry shampoo as a temporary measure instead.

Dry shampoos come in powder form and it's essential that they are brushed out thoroughly after use or they'll leave your scalp dry and itchy and your hair looking dull. Once you've put the powder on as instructed, spend a minute or so brushing it out. You can also use ordinary talc as an emergency alternative.

Watchpoint

Never use your fingernails when massaging in shampoo or you could scratch your scalp.

IT JUST WON'T WASH

It is possible to leave your hair unwashed for ages and for it to still look perfectly allright. But first you need to consider your hair type and whether you can face each day, without having washed your hair.

Still, if you'd like to have a go at leaving your hair unwashed for a while, first look at your hair type. This idea works best on coarse, dry and wavy hair – fine, greasy hair doesn't look too good if left unwashed.

It may sound hard to believe but you can get away with simply massaging a little conditioner into your scalp when you feel your hair is dirty and then rinsing it away with water.

You'll also need to brush hair more regularly so you can draw oil away from the roots and loosen any dead hair.

If you decide to experiment with leaving your hair unwashed for a while, good luck, but if you find it's not working for you and your hair looks absolutely dreadful, this can be easily remedied – all you need to do is reach for the shampoo and wash your hair!

ON THE FRINGE

A precisely cut fringe starts to lose its shape when your hair grows. Take up DIY trimming and bring your fringe back into line with a few short snips!

BLUNT CUTS create...

bold looks that show off both your hair and features.

They suit:
● Strong hair colours – such as red, dark brown and golden blonde.
● Straight, thick hair – they will emphasise the texture and condition.
● Sculptured, fine features.
● One-length hair – from a bob to waist-length!

TEXTURED FRINGES create...

soft, romantic looks that gently frame your features.

They suit:
● Softer hair colours – dark blondes and mid-browns.
● Highlighted hair – the layers emphasise the colour.
● Hair that's growing out a colour or a perm – textured hair hides any strong contrast between the roots and main length.
● Layered and curly hair.
● Fine hair – texture adds body.
● Soft, rounded features.

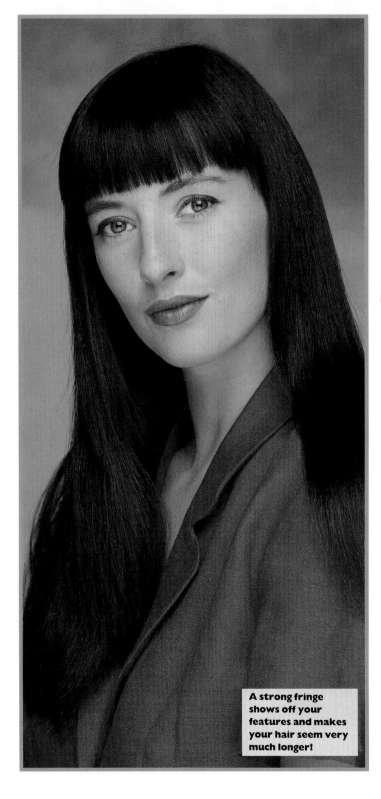

A strong fringe shows off your features and makes your hair seem very much longer!

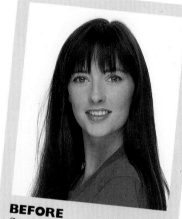

BEFORE
Start with freshly washed and dried hair. Don't use styling products since they can cause your hair to curl slightly.

GOING STRAIGHT

Show off long, shiny hair and fine features with a blunt-cut fringe.

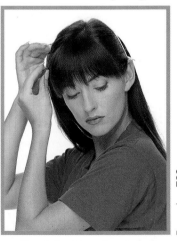

Brown top: ZOO

1 *Comb the fringe forwards then clip the rest of your hair out of the way so you can't cut into it by accident.*

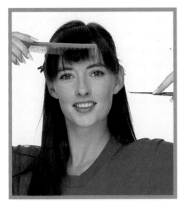

2 Comb your fringe down flat so that you can cut your hair to an even length. To find the correct line for your fringe measure from a point halfway back to the centre of your crown and out to the edges of each eyebrow. Start trimming, with short, neat snips, at the centre of your fringe so that you've a guideline for both sides.

Cut your fringe when it is damp or towel-dried since wet hair hangs lower on your face.

Tip

Look straight ahead into a mirror to see what you are doing. Don't look up because you'll lift your eyebrows and make your fringe look much longer than it really is!

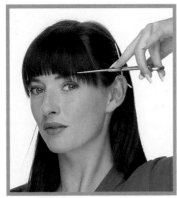

3 Comb your fringe down after each cut to make sure the hair is flat for the next snip. Move round to the side of your fringe and trim this too.

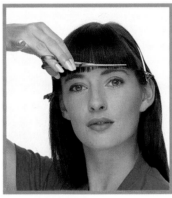

4 Use the original centre length as a guide when you trim the other side. Then tidy up any long, straggly hairs – but go easy or you could end up with less fringe than you'd bargained for!

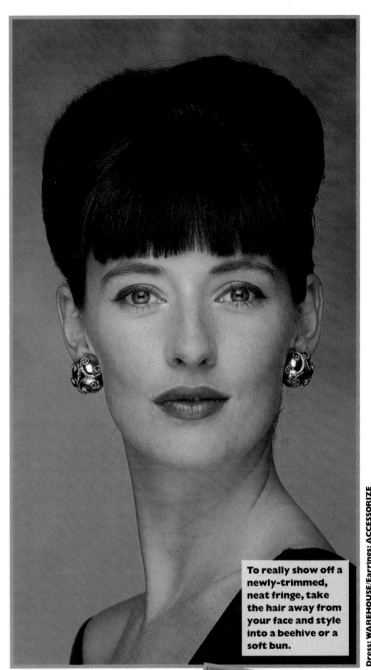

To really show off a newly-trimmed, neat fringe, take the hair away from your face and style into a beehive or a soft bun.

Dress: WAREHOUSE/Earrings: ACCESSORIZE

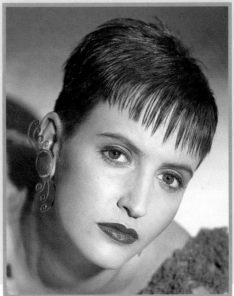

BRIGHT LIGHTS This fringe is only slightly shorter than the bob.
SUITS: Medium to thick hair.

SCHWARZKOPF

CLYNOL

IN TRIM A short wispy fringe softens this otherwise severe crop and emphasises eyes and eyebrow shape.
SUITS: Fine to medium thick, layered hair.

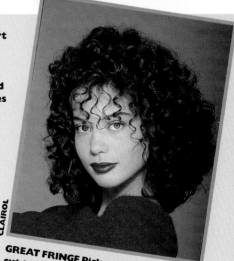

CLAIROL

GREAT FRINGE Pick a few tendrils and cut to eyebrow length.
SUITS: Curly hair.

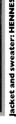
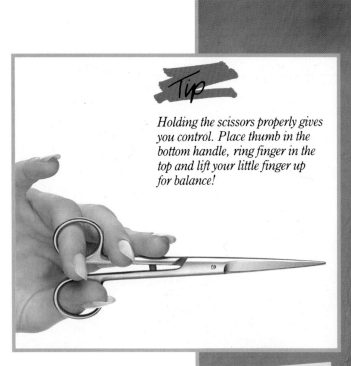

SOFT TOUCH

As a change from a straight fringe, try layering it for a much softer and more versatile finish. You won't lose out on its thickness.

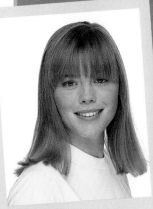

BEFORE
Make sure that your hair is dry and well-combed before you begin.

A layered fringe softens your features. Its thicker texture adds volume and weight to your hair.

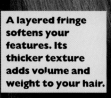

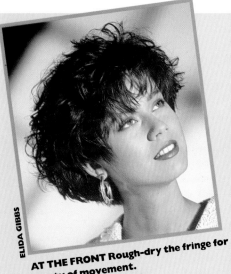

ELIDA GIBBS

AT THE FRONT Rough-dry the fringe for plenty of movement.
SUITS: Thick, curly hair.

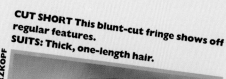

CUT SHORT This blunt-cut fringe shows off regular features.
SUITS: Thick, one-length hair.

SCHWARZKOPF

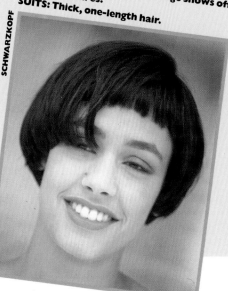

L'ORÉAL

FRINGE FRIENDS Team up with your man and have matching fringes for double the style!
SUITS: Thick-textured hair with a wave.

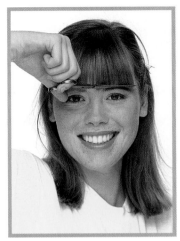

1 *Carefully trim your fringe so it's level with your eyebrows. Layering will shorten it to the right length.*

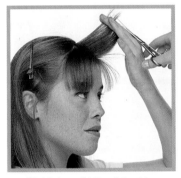

2 *Hold the middle of the fringe at the ends and pull it up vertically. The shorter hair will fall forwards, leaving the longer length free. Trim this, from front to back, along your fingers – use this as a guide and trim the rest to match.*

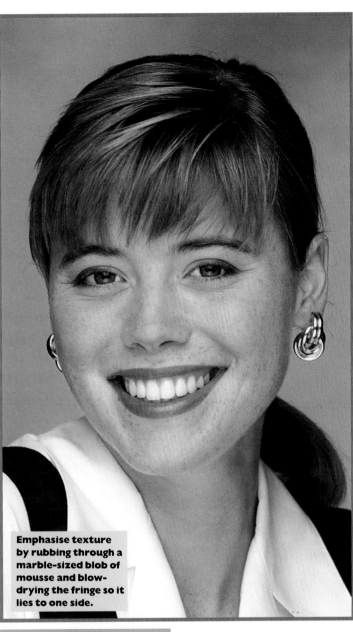

Emphasise texture by rubbing through a marble-sized blob of mousse and blow-drying the fringe so it lies to one side.

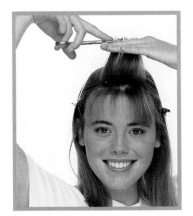

3 *To check the fringe is straight, lift it up widthways. Hold the hair at the ends so that the shorter lengths fall forward. The line across the longer hair should be even, but trim lightly if not.*

4 *Finally, to soften the bottom of your fringe, snip vertically along the edge. Aim to reach 2.5 cm/1 in into the fringe length.*

Photographs: PAUL LAWRENCE/Make-up: LIZZIE COURT/Hair: JUSTIN WILLIAMS/Pinafore and shirt: WAREHOUSE/Earrings: ACCESSORIZE

FRINGE BENEFITS

ON WET HAIR

● Work a pea-sized blob of gel into the roots of your fringe to spike it up high.
● Rub a marble-sized blob of mousse into the fringe and blow-dry for texture.
● Thickening lotion adds weight.
● Blow-dry your fringe straight, brushing with a round brush. For a solid look use heated straighteners.

ON DRY HAIR

● Tease a thumbnail-sized blob of wax through your fringe to break up the volume slightly, or smooth it down the length for a solid look.
● Spritz with hairspray to create a soft flick.
● Gently back-comb the roots for height and extra volume.
● Comb through a pea-sized blob of wet-look gel for a really slick finish.

Naturally curly or tightly permed hair looks great with a fringe. Go for a layered fringe, or just a few strands or tendrils rather than a thick, heavy, blunt-cut, fringe.

FRINGE FACTS

● When 'Beatle fringes' were popular in the Sixties, there was an outbreak of spots on foreheads! Don't let this happen to you – always keep your fringe scrupulously clean.
● A shorter fringe makes your face look wider and rounder. A longer fringe will give length to your face.
● Don't let your fringe hang below your eyebrows all the time. Your hair could look untidy and you risk straining your eyes!
● A slightly curved fringe flatters a long nose or a small face.

No time to wash your hair? Then wash just your fringe instead and let it dry naturally – a clean fringe will instantly pep up lank hair.

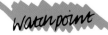

If your parting's on the left, the left-hand side of your fringe may be slightly longer, with the reverse effect if your parting is on the right. Trim to even it up.

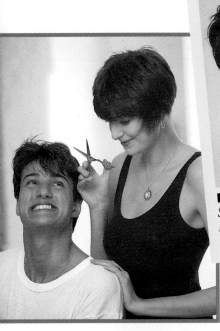

BEFORE
Suggest he washes his hair first, or damp it down with a water spray.

GIVE HIM A TRIM

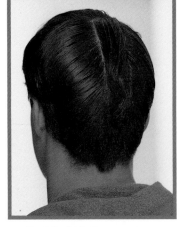

1 *Part the hair from ear to ear. Next, make two partings down the back of the head, dividing the back hair into three panels.*

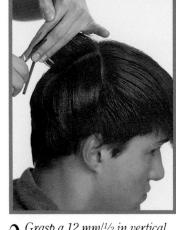

2 *Grasp a 12 mm/½ in vertical section from the top of the centre panel between your middle and index fingers, then cut.*

For most men a trip to the hairdresser or barber is a bit of a chore, however much their hair may be in need of a trim. So why not trim it yourself – it's quite easy once you know how. Although you won't be able to manage a complete restyle – that's best left to the professionals – you can certainly give him a tidier look.

Make sure you've got plenty of time to spare – even a trim can't be rushed if you're not an expert. You'll also need a sharp pair of hairdressing scissors and, most important, a co-operative man with confidence in your ability. After all, his hair is in your hands!

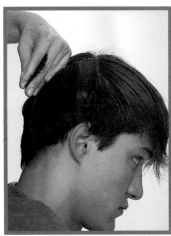

3 *Now take the next section down in the same centre panel and cut it in the same way. Continue cutting downwards.*

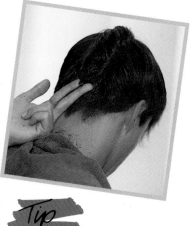

Tip

To keep your hand steady when cutting the last section at the nape of the neck, rest your knuckles against his neck.

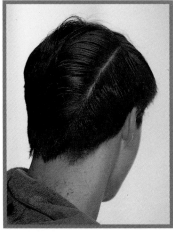

4 *Make another parting 4 cm/1½ in away from the previous one. Starting with the section nearest the crown, cut as before.*

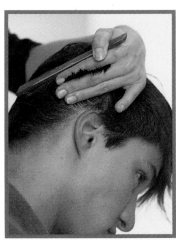

5 *Now cut the section nearest the ears. Once you've completed one side of the head, cut the other in the same way.*

Photographs: STEVE SMITH/Hair: PENNY ATTWOOD/Make-up: ELLIE LEBLANC

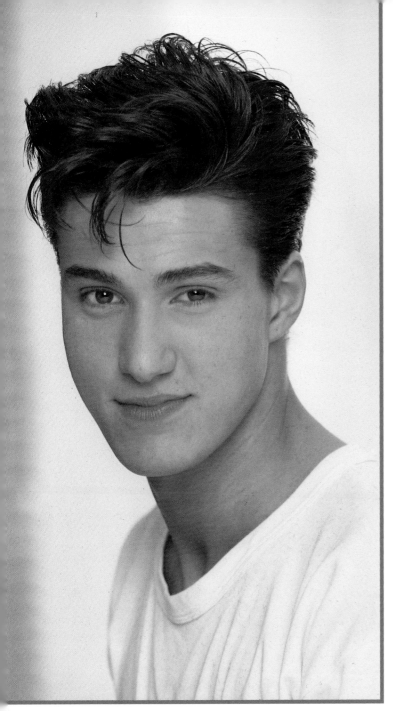

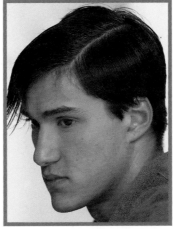

8 *Make a further parting 4 cm/ 1½ in away from the previous one. Cut this section in the same way as step 7.*

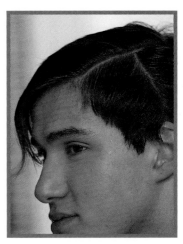

9 *Make a vertical parting starting just above the ears to meet the previous parting.*

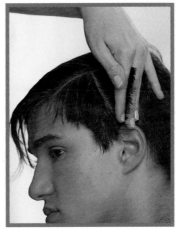

10 *Cut the back section then the front, angling your fingers downwards. Repeat steps 8 and 9 on the other side of the head.*

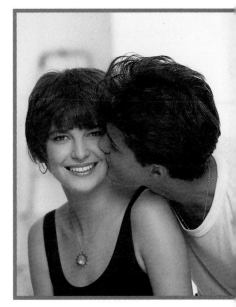

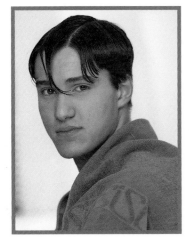

6 *To cut the front, make two partings down the centre in the same way as the back. You now have three front panels..*

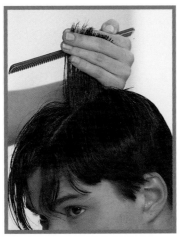

7 *Cut the centre panel starting at the crown. Lift the hair upwards and cut at an angle to give a heavy fringe.*

TRIMMING TIPS

● **Make sure you read through our guide thoroughly before you start.** It's a good idea to run through the steps first without using scissors.
● **Don't use any old scissors** which come to hand. It's worth investing in a pair of hairdressing scissors to do the job properly. You'll find them in most major chemists.
● **Sit your man in a chair** that's the right height for you to cut his hair comfortably.
● **Keep a water-spray handy** to keep the hair damp as you cut. You'll find it's much easier for

cutting a straight line.
● **Put a towel around his shoulders** to catch the drips and snips as you cut.
● **As a guide when you cut a new section of hair,** include a few strands of hair from the previous one, so you can match the length.
● **Comb through the section of hair** before you cut so that it's smooth and tangle-free.
● **Use hair clips** if hair's long, or it won't stay out of the way.
● **Wet shave the nape of his neck** if straggly hairs are spoiling the finished hairline.

CUTTING KIDS' HAIR

If your little brother or sister's in need of a trim but you know that a trip to the hairdresser will end in tears, why not have a go yourself? Learn basic cutting and you'll keep any tearaway tidy

Trimming a child's hair at home isn't as hard as it sounds. Once a good basic cut has been established – and a hairdresser really does have to do this – trimming it back into shape is easy. Hair needs to be neatened up every six to eight weeks, so alternate a home trim with a trip to the salon. Never try to attempt a complete re-style – this is completely different to a trim and should be left to the professionals. Just put on a favourite TV programme to distract the child and away you go!

You need:
towel
comb
water spray
section clips
scissors
hairdryer
brush
gel

SCISSOR TALK

Buy a pair of *hairdressing* scissors with slightly rounded ends as these are safest for children's hair. To hold the scissors, put your thumb in the handle of the top blade, and your third finger in the handle of the bottom blade. Keeping the bottom blade still, cut with the thumb blade. Take short snips closing the blades together each time. Use only the ends of the blades to cut.

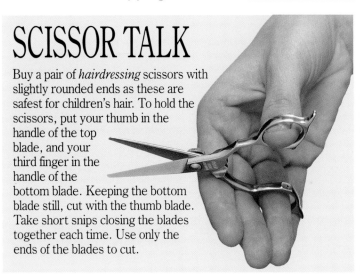

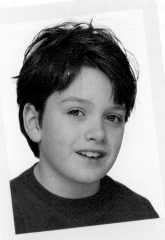

BEFORE
Hair is definitely in need of a good trim!

TRIMMING LAYERS

The simplest way to tidy up a layered cut is to start by trimming around the hairline first, then go on to trim the layers.

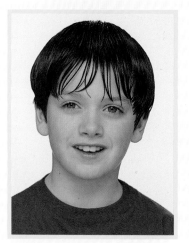

1 *Wash and towel-dry the hair, then comb it forwards from the crown and down at the sides and back.*

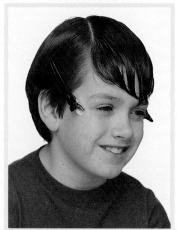

2 *Part the hair from just above the temples right back to the centre of the crown. Clip the rest of the hair out of the way.*

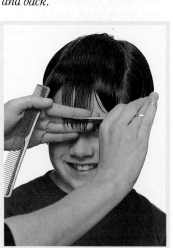

3 *Comb the fringe forwards, then take a section in the centre and cut a straight line in precise snips.*

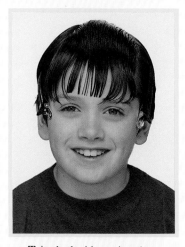

4 *Trim both sides using the centre line as a guide. Make the fringe curve slightly downwards at the ends.*

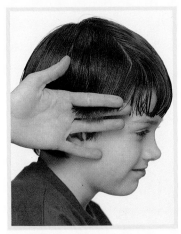

5 Trim the sides to the same length as the fringe until you reach the top of the ear.

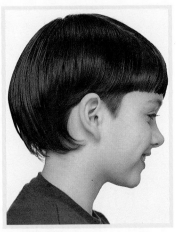

6 Comb the hair downwards in front of the ear and trim to form a neat triangle shape.

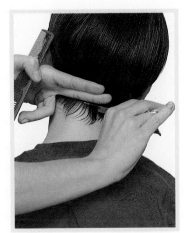

7 For the back, comb hair straight down, then rest the bottom blade against the neck. Start in the centre and snip towards sides.

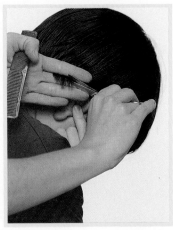

8 Trim back corners. Comb hair downwards and continue cutting along the same line, curving slightly up above ears.

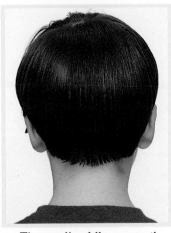

9 The napeline follows a gentle curve which suits a young child. For a sharper line, trim sides at a steeper angle.

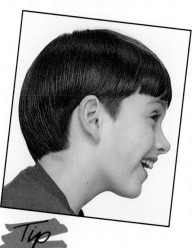

Tip

Don't worry if the hair looks solid, the layers you are about to add will soften it.

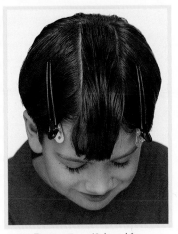

10 Part a 5 cm/2 in wide section along the top of the head and comb forwards. Clip the sides out of the way.

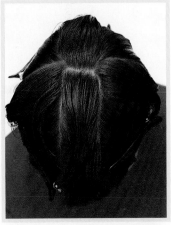

11 Section the hair again, this time from the crown to either side of the ears. Section the back hair to the nape.

TRIM TIPS

● Before cutting, go through the steps without scissors to feel how the hair lies.

● Hair looks shorter when it dries, so cut the fringe slightly longer than you want.

● Always hold a cut section and a long section together as you trim so that you get an even result.

● Trim layers to the same length by holding the hair at 90° to the head.

● Make sure the child is sitting up straight while you cut back hair or you may end up with a wavy line!

● Get the child to hold the top of his ear down while you trim above it.

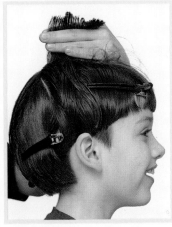

12 Trim the first section from crown to fringe, lifting the hair in vertical sections.

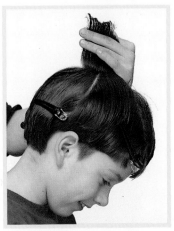

13 Continue trimming this middle section in equal stages down to the nape of the neck.

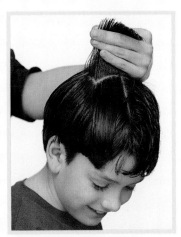

14 Now, holding the hair vertically in your fingers, trim straight across the ear to ear section.

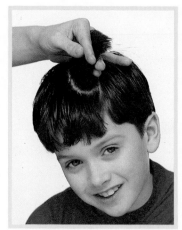

15 *Make a diagonal section from the crown out to the hairline and trim. Repeat in sections around the head.*

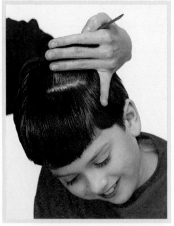

16 *Now check your cutting! Dry hair and lift a few sections across the head. If it's not all the same length, trim to even up.*

DO'S and DONT'S

- Never cut hair in a hurry.
- Always cut hair in a good light so that you can see exactly what you're doing.
- Keep a spray of lukewarm water handy to dampen the hair if it begins to dry out.

- When cutting a fringe, hold the hair between your fingers with the finger underneath resting on the child's forehead. This will reassure the child that you are between him and the scissors!

TRIMMING ONE LENGTH HAIR

Whether you take off an inch or three inches the steps are the same. Allow about 45 minutes to do the job properly.

FINISHED
Blow-dry or add a little gel for a casual, spiky look.

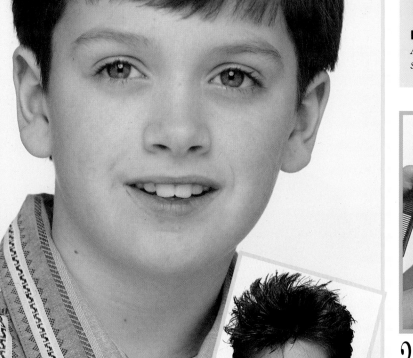

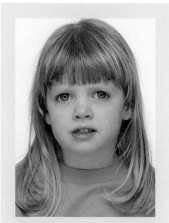

BEFORE
A one-length cut that hasn't seen scissors for six months!

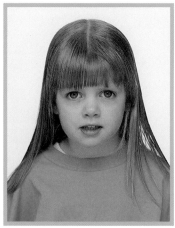

1 *Start by washing and towel-drying the hair. Comb it straight down then part neatly in the centre.*

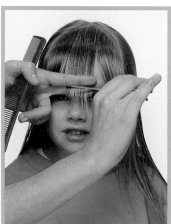

2 *Where the hair recedes above the temples, part the hair back to the crown. Take the centre section and trim across.*

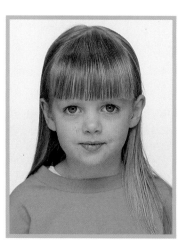

3 *Use this first section as a guide for trimming both sides of the fringe level. Comb the fringe down and snip off any stray hairs.*

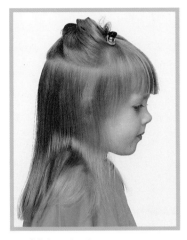

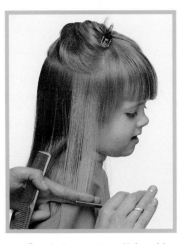

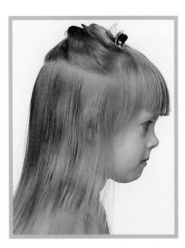

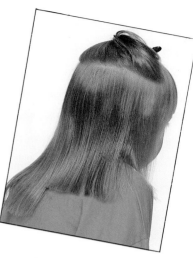

4 Make a horizontal parting around the top of the child's head, then clip the top section out of the way.

5 Comb down a 5 cm/2 in wide section of hair. Hold it between two fingers and trim along the underside taking small snips.

6 Continue trimming all the way round cutting along the same line. Try not to lift the hair or you'll lose the line.

Tip Take a few steps back every now and then to double-check that you're still cutting a straight line.

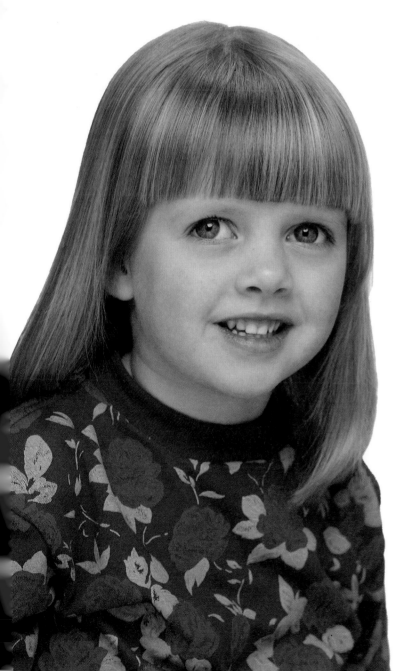

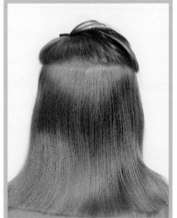

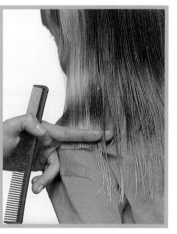

7 When you've finished trimming the underneath section it should be one even length. Trim any stray hairs.

8 Take down the top section of hair and comb through. Trim to the same length as the underneath section.

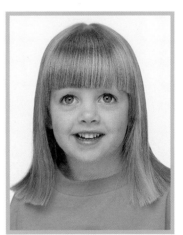

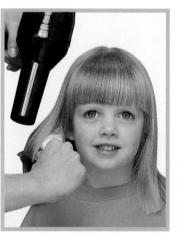

9 The finished cut looking nice and neat after 6.5 cm/2½ in have been cut away.

10 While the hair is still damp, blow-dry the ends under using a round brush to soften the line.

Photographs: ALISTAIR HUGHES/Hair: PENNY ATTWOOD/Boy's shirt and T-shirt: NEXT BOYS and GIRLS/Girl's T-shirt: BENETTON

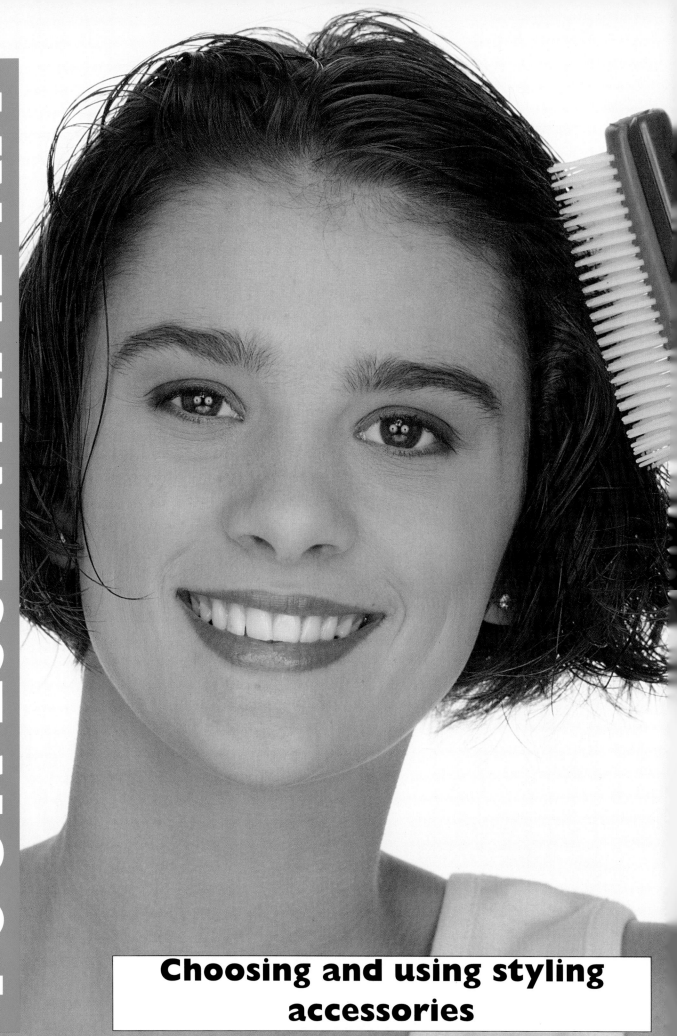

YOUR ESSENTIAL KIT

Choosing and using styling accessories

THE HEAT IS ON

Don't be a hothead and buy the first hairdryer you set eyes on. Most of us only own one so it's worth finding out which dryer is right for your style. Get switched on with our guide to what's on offer

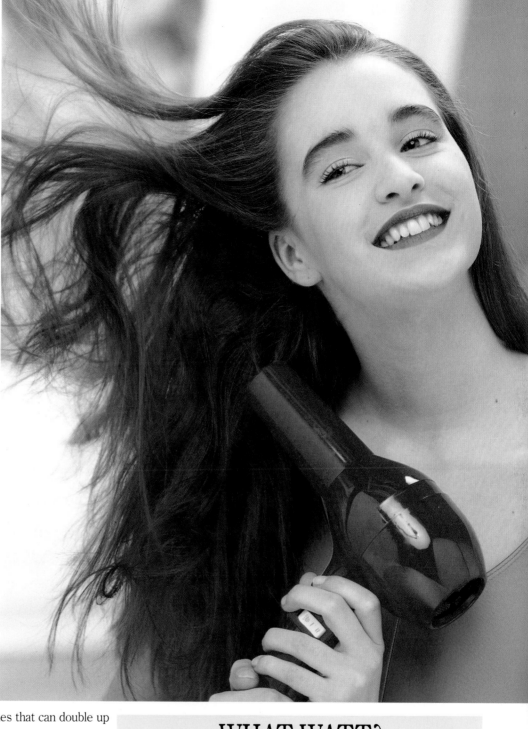

One hairdryer may look pretty much like another and you may think that the only difference is in its colour or size. But hairdryers do have an amazing range of features and functions.

You'll find dryers with different speed and heat settings and a range of nozzles to suit a variety of styling techniques. They also come in various sizes. There's a number of mini-sized dryers you can take on holiday, larger professional-style ones – just like those your hairdresser uses, dryers that make very little noise

and even ones that can double up as an iron!

Think carefully about what you actually want from your hairdryer before you part with your money. Will it suit your hair type? Is it the best one for making the most of your particular style? Is it small enough to fit in your suitcase and so on?

Make sure you know exactly what you're buying by reading the details on the back of the box, or the best way of all is to get a shop assistant to show you what is available.

WHAT WATT?

One of the most important things when buying a hairdryer is to check that the wattage (the amount of power) will suit your styling requirements. Most dryers are around 1200 watts on their highest setting but when switched to different levels of heat and speeds may be as low as 600-800 watts. Use the coolest, lowest speeds for fixing curls and setting your style and for drying permed or naturally curly hair.

The fastest, most powerful dryers are the professional type and these are around 1600/2000 watts. These dryers are great if you want to dry your hair quickly or your hair is long and thick. However, do take care not to use your dryer on its highest setting too often as this can damage your hair.

Travel dryers usually have a low wattage (600-800 watts). These are only suitable for holidays as they tend not to have enough power for everyday use.

DRYER ROUND-UP

Check out all types of different dryers and their special features.

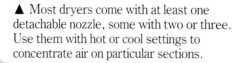

▲ Most dryers come with at least one detachable nozzle, some with two or three. Use them with hot or cool settings to concentrate air on particular sections.
Good for: styling small areas such as a fringe or creating small curls.

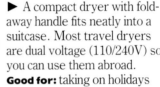

▶ A compact dryer with fold-away handle fits neatly into a suitcase. Most travel dryers are dual voltage (110/240V) so you can use them abroad.
Good for: taking on holidays and weekends away.

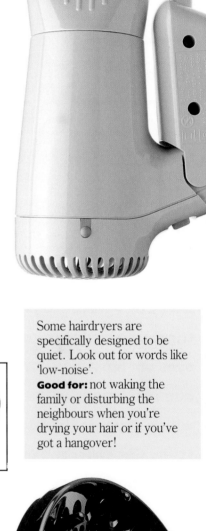

Watch point

Never use your hairdryer in the bathroom or anywhere it is likely to come into contact with liquid.

▶ A dryer with a cool setting feature. Switching from hot to cool during styling will help set your hair into shape.
Good for: fixing waves and curls, putting the shape back into a perm and generally creating long-lasting styles.

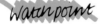

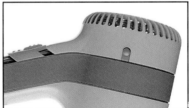

▲ **Anti-skid pads – on the sides of dryers stop them scratching and sliding off table tops.**

Some hairdryers are specifically designed to be quiet. Look out for words like 'low-noise'.
Good for: not waking the family or disturbing the neighbours when you're drying your hair or if you've got a hangover!

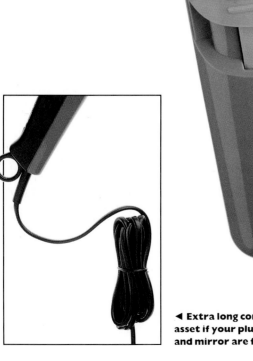

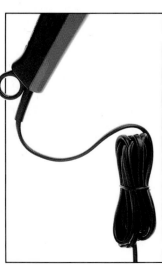

◀ **Extra long cord – an asset if your plug socket and mirror are far apart.**

▶ A diffuser is a dish-shaped attachment with prongs that you attach to the nozzle end of your dryer. It enables the air from the dryer to circulate over a wider area and is great for separating curls. It also stops your hair from drying out or frizzing.
Good for: permed and naturally wavy or curly styles.

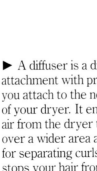

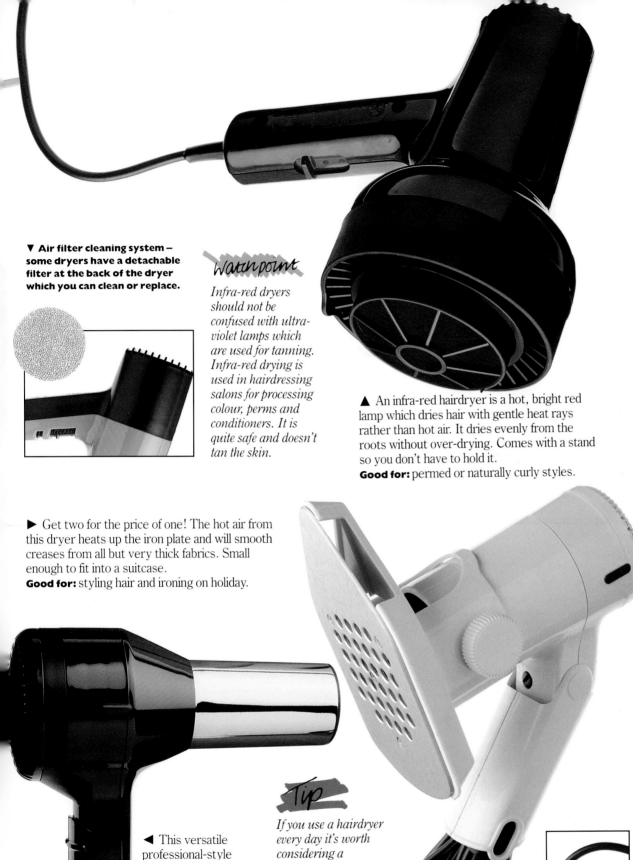

▼ **Air filter cleaning system –** some dryers have a detachable filter at the back of the dryer which you can clean or replace.

Infra-red dryers should not be confused with ultra-violet lamps which are used for tanning. Infra-red drying is used in hairdressing salons for processing colour, perms and conditioners. It is quite safe and doesn't tan the skin.

▲ An infra-red hairdryer is a hot, bright red lamp which dries hair with gentle heat rays rather than hot air. It dries evenly from the roots without over-drying. Comes with a stand so you don't have to hold it.
Good for: permed or naturally curly styles.

▶ Get two for the price of one! The hot air from this dryer heats up the iron plate and will smooth creases from all but very thick fabrics. Small enough to fit into a suitcase.
Good for: styling hair and ironing on holiday.

◀ This versatile professional-style dryer has a slim nozzle for concentrated drying. It's also lightweight.
Good for: general drying and it is especially useful if you want to blow-dry your hair straight.

Tip

If you use a hairdryer every day it's worth considering a 'professional' dryer. These are designed to withstand the rigours of continuous drying in a hairdressing salon, but they are easily obtainable for home use and should last twice as long as ordinary dryers.

▶ **Hang-up loop –** useful if you want to store your dryer neatly.

SOME LIKE IT HOT

● *Always towel-dry your hair before you start blow-drying. If it's soaking wet you'll have to use the dryer for longer and you'll run the risk of damaging your hair.*

● *Never have the setting too hot and always try to hold the dryer at least 15 cm/ 6 in away from your hair – any closer and you could burn your hair. The exception to this rule is when you're using a diffuser attachment, which is specially designed to work close to your head.*

● *Make sure you keep the dryer moving constantly. Don't concentrate the heat on one area of hair for more than a couple of seconds at a time.*

● *First of all, rough dry your hair on a fast speed without a nozzle. Once your hair feels about half dry, switch to a slower speed then put on a nozzle for more controlled styling.*

● *Make sure your hair is completely dry, right through to the roots. If it's even slightly damp your hair will flop.*

● *Occasionally clean the mesh or vent at the back of your dryer where dust collects and replace the filter if it's removable.*

Photographs: ADRIAN TAYLOR

33

Don't let styling your hair be a drag! Comb through our essential guide and get kitted out with the right tools for taming your hair

COMB ON

A comb is such a basic bit of hair-care equipment that you probably use one every day and never give it a second thought. But, in fact, a comb can be an invaluable styling aid. You can use it for back-combing, blow-drying, lifting curls, making partings and for sectioning when you're winding your hair up in rollers.

In order to get the most from your style you'll probably need two or three different combs. One with widely-spaced teeth to use when your hair is wet, a tailcomb for making sections or partings, and a fine-toothed comb that you can use for back-combing when you want to add body.

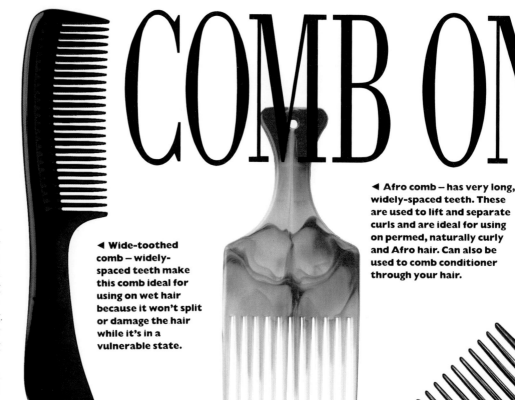

◄ **Wide-toothed comb** – widely-spaced teeth make this comb ideal for using on wet hair because it won't split or damage the hair while it's in a vulnerable state.

◄ **Afro comb** – has very long, widely-spaced teeth. These are used to lift and separate curls and are ideal for using on permed, naturally curly and Afro hair. Can also be used to comb conditioner through your hair.

COMB TALK

● Natural materials like horn or tortoiseshell tend to be quite expensive, but are best for your hair because they don't create static.

● Avoid metal combs (these are very difficult to find these days because they are known to be so bad for your hair).

● Never use an old comb with sharp or jagged edges – since it will split and damage hair.

● Keep combs clean. Wash them frequently in warm soapy water, rinse, and leave to dry naturally.

● Be gentle when you're using a comb, especially if hair is wet.

● Move a comb down the length of your hair from the roots to the ends and then there's no reason why your style shouldn't comb up trumps!

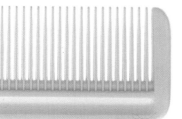

▲ **Mousse comb** – looks like a flat brush with two rows of teeth. Use it to distribute mousse or other styling products evenly through your hair – always combing from the roots through to the ends.

▲ **Baby comb** – specially designed to use on very fine, baby hair. It has softly rounded teeth that won't scratch or damage a delicate scalp.

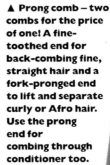

▲ **Prong comb** – two combs for the price of one! A fine-toothed end for back-combing fine, straight hair and a fork-pronged end to lift and separate curly or Afro hair. Use the prong end for combing through conditioner too.

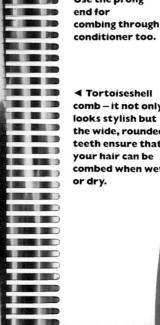

◄ **Tortoiseshell comb** – it not only looks stylish but the wide, rounded teeth ensure that your hair can be combed when wet or dry.

KENT

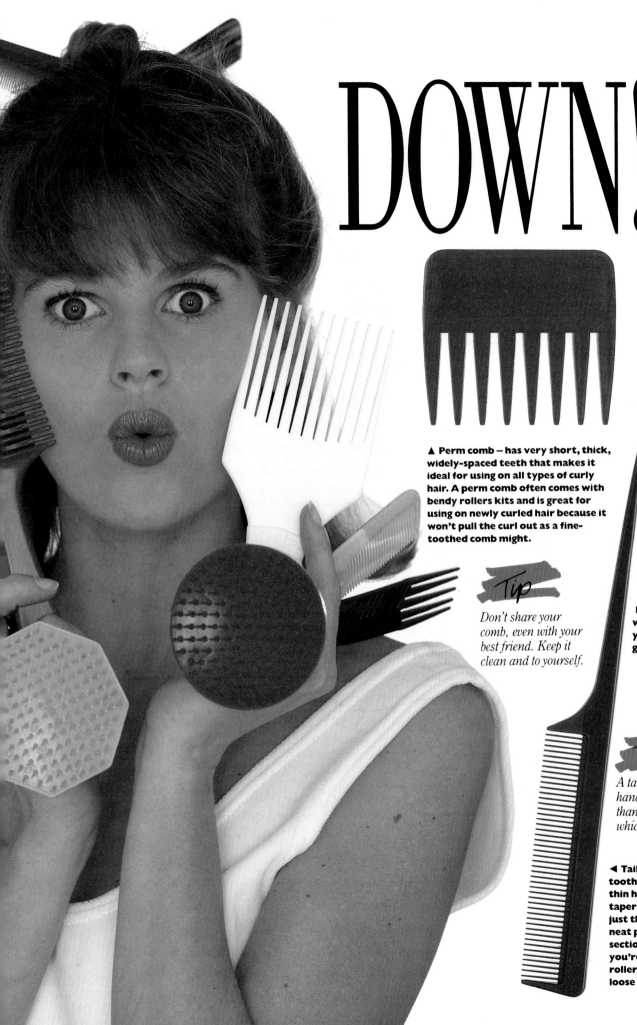

DOWN!

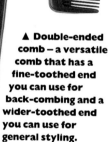

▲ Perm comb – has very short, thick, widely-spaced teeth that makes it ideal for using on all types of curly hair. A perm comb often comes with bendy rollers kits and is great for using on newly curled hair because it won't pull the curl out as a fine-toothed comb might.

Tip

Don't share your comb, even with your best friend. Keep it clean and to yourself.

▲ Double-ended comb – a versatile comb that has a fine-toothed end you can use for back-combing and a wider-toothed end you can use for general styling.

Tip

A tailcomb with a metal handle will last longer than a plastic one – which can break easily.

◄ Tailcomb – a fine-toothed comb with a long thin handle that generally tapers down to a point. It's just the thing for making neat partings, picking out sections of hair when you're winding it up into rollers, or tucking in any loose ends.

Main picture: NICK COLE/Still-life: ADRIAN TAYLOR

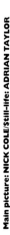

HEAT WAVE

Try out a hot brush and warm to curls and waves at the flick of a switch. You'll transform your hair into a great new style in a matter of minutes

LOOSE WAVES

Tousled waves on one-length hair

1 Your hair should be dry and tangle free. Use the larger bristles on the brush for a loose wave.

2 To create ringlets, separate your hair into 5 cm/2 in wide vertical sections. Wrap each section, in turn, around the barrel to within 2.5 cm/1 in of your head, winding along the length of the barrel so you end up with a roll shape.

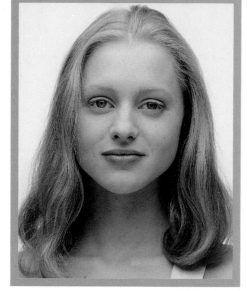

Tip

Fill the steam reservoir with water and heat the brush until the light comes on. Wind the hair up around the brush and press the cap once to release the steam.

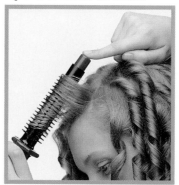

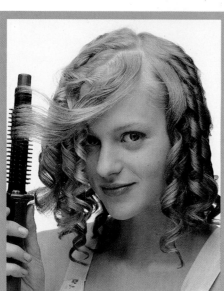

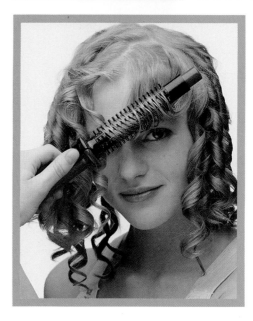

WHAT'S WHAT

Hot brushes are available in several different barrel sizes. The length and density of the bristles can also vary.

Some of the latest models have interchangeable bristles to make the brush suitable for all types of hair. Here's a guide to what will give the best results.

Choose larger bristles for:
● Big, loose curls.
● Hair below shoulder length.
● Adding body to long hair.

Choose small bristles for:
● Small tight curls.
● Short hair.
● Adding body to short hair.

If your hot brush doesn't have a choice of bristles, take smaller sections of hair to make smaller curls, and wider sections for soft, body-giving waves.

Steam heat
The steam release button gives out a measured burst of steam each time you press it. You don't need to press it more than once for each curl.

If your hot brush doesn't have steam then hold the curl for slightly longer to give it a chance to set properly.

3 Hold the brush in place for about 30 seconds. If your hair holds a curl easily then leave it for a shorter time, if it doesn't, hold it for up to a minute. Press the curl release button and draw the brush away from your hair so that it unwinds. The curl should be tight and springy.

THE RIGHT BRUSH

Need a new hairbrush? There's such a big variety available now that trying to find the most suitable one for you can leave you bristling with emotion! We go through the types available with a fine tooth comb

It's easy to get confused by all the shapes when you go into your local chemist shop to buy a new brush. But they haven't just been designed as accessories to clutter up your dressing table, brushes do all have special functions.

Generally speaking, brushes fall into two categories – there are brushes like an ordinary hairbrush that are ideal for general grooming or brushing, and then there are the more specialised brushes like the vent brush which you use for styling your hair with the help of a hairdryer.

BRUSH WORK

You probably possess a brush of one sort or another, but chances are you haven't kept it in tip-top condition. It may have half the bristles missing, or be dirty, or it may just have suffered years of neglect and be in a rather shabby and battered state like a favourite old teddy bear.

But whatever state the brush or brushes you have are in, you must get a good general brush that suits the texture and length of your hair. It should be made of bristles that are right for your hair type (either nylon, natural bristle, a mixture of the two or plastic).

It's no use buying the most expensive hogs' hairbrush on the market if a nylon one will suit you better. Bear in mind that **natural bristle** brushes are best suited to long straight or fine long hair. The natural bristles will help your hair to look sleek and shiny without damaging the scalp. They will also help to calm down the static electricity in your hair which is likely to make it flyaway and difficult to manage.

A **nylon and bristle mix brush** will suit you best if your hair is thick and wavy and a **nylon brush** suits most hair types and textures but is particularly good for short hair.

Vent brushes are simply brushes that have widely-spaced bristles or quills, and air vents to allow the hot air from your dryer to circulate and prevent your hair over-heating.

Vent brushes come in cylindrical shapes or the more common rectangular shape. The cylindrical brush works best if you have got short or mid-length hair that's a medium to thick texture. You can use it for curling your hair under or straightening it.

Simply divide your hair into sections when blow-drying, being careful not to pull the hair too tightly near the tip of the brush as it is likely to get all tangled up. Direct the heat from your dryer from roots to ends – the quills all the way round the brush should allow you to get a good tension on the hair to straighten it or curl it under. Allow each section to dry thoroughly before carefully removing the brush.

Flat vent brushes are great for getting natural, free-flowing effects. They are very useful if your hair has slight wave or curl because the waves will not be dragged out and pulled straight as they would be with a more traditional type of brush.

You will probably have seen **bobble-tipped** brushes in the shops. Sometimes called wet brushes, the purpose of these (often very brightly coloured) bobbly ends is to protect your hair – they won't pull it, they won't scratch your scalp and they can be used to very gently brush the tangles out of wet hair.

They are also used for general brushing and blow-drying looser styles and suit most lengths of hair except very short. Bobble-ended brushes work best on hair that is medium thick through to hair which is very thick.

Radial brushes are round styling brushes that are usually either plastic or a nylon and bristle mixture. These can be used to create curls on all lengths of hair and for adding style and shape to short hair.

If your hair is short and wavy use a radial brush for flicking back unruly fringes, for creating gentle curls or waves, or simply for styling.

Shampoo brush – this is excellent for gently massaging your scalp when you're shampooing. It works well on a dry scalp.

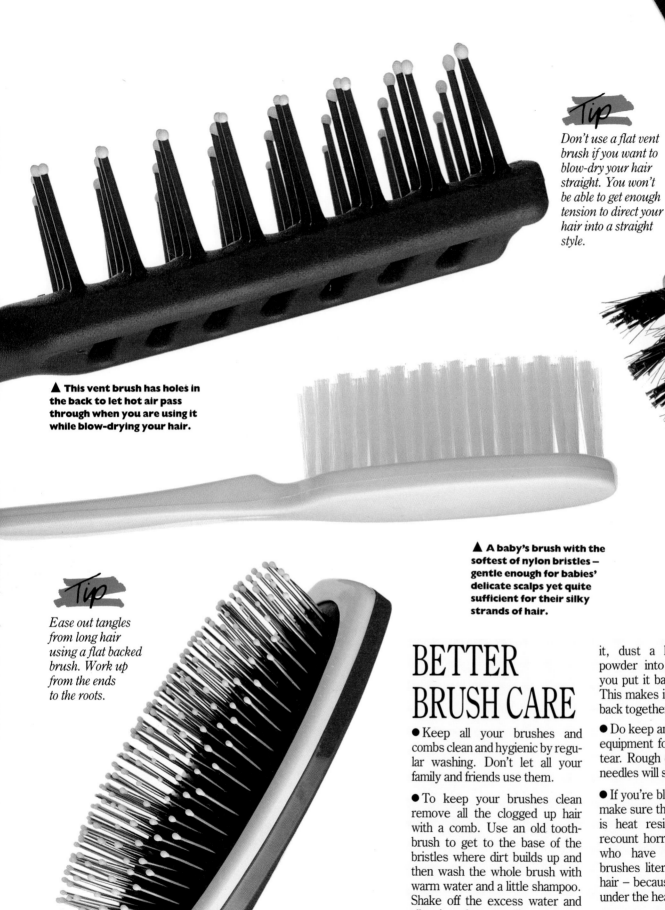

▲ This vent brush has holes in the back to let hot air pass through when you are using it while blow-drying your hair.

Tip

Don't use a flat vent brush if you want to blow-dry your hair straight. You won't be able to get enough tension to direct your hair into a straight style.

▲ A baby's brush with the softest of nylon bristles — gentle enough for babies' delicate scalps yet quite sufficient for their silky strands of hair.

▶ A thickly-bristled styling brush, ideal for creating waves and flicks.

Tip

Ease out tangles from long hair using a flat backed brush. Work up from the ends to the roots.

◀ A bobble-tipped brush (wet brush) — the bobbles mean it can be safely used on wet hair.

BETTER BRUSH CARE

● Keep all your brushes and combs clean and hygienic by regular washing. Don't let all your family and friends use them.

● To keep your brushes clean remove all the clogged up hair with a comb. Use an old toothbrush to get to the base of the bristles where dirt builds up and then wash the whole brush with warm water and a little shampoo. Shake off the excess water and allow it to dry naturally.

● If you have one of those brushes that you can pull the rubber-cushioned bit out to clean it, dust a little bit of talcum powder into the runners when you put it back in after cleaning. This makes it much easier to put back together.

● Do keep an eye on all your hair equipment for signs of wear and tear. Rough edges or split quills/needles will split your hair.

● If you're blow-drying your hair, make sure the brush you're using is heat resistant. Hairdressers recount horror stories of people who have come in to have brushes literally cut out of their hair — because they have melted under the heat of the hairdryer.

● Use your hairdryer on a moderate heat, not a fierce heat. Your brush will last much longer and so will your hair!

Photographs: ADRIAN TAYLOR

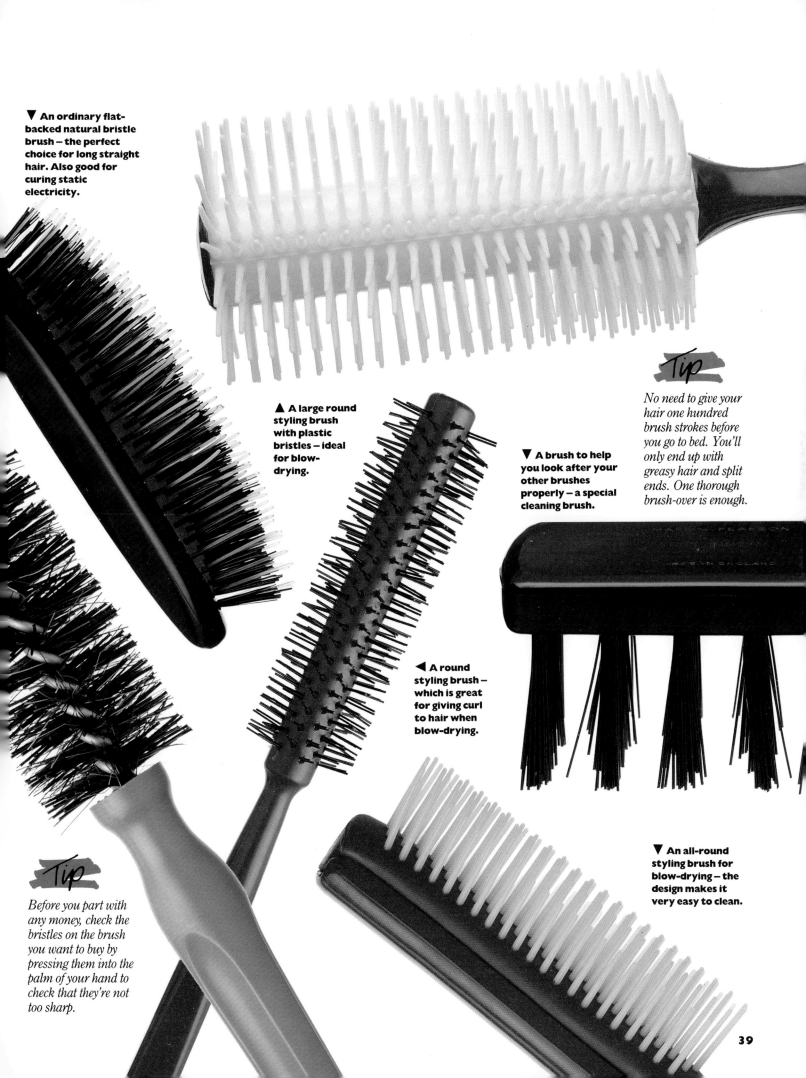

▼ An ordinary flat-backed natural bristle brush – the perfect choice for long straight hair. Also good for curing static electricity.

▲ A large round styling brush with plastic bristles – ideal for blow-drying.

▼ A brush to help you look after your other brushes properly – a special cleaning brush.

◀ A round styling brush – which is great for giving curl to hair when blow-drying.

▼ An all-round styling brush for blow-drying – the design makes it very easy to clean.

Tip

No need to give your hair one hundred brush strokes before you go to bed. You'll only end up with greasy hair and split ends. One thorough brush-over is enough.

Tip

Before you part with any money, check the bristles on the brush you want to buy by pressing them into the palm of your hand to check that they're not too sharp.

39

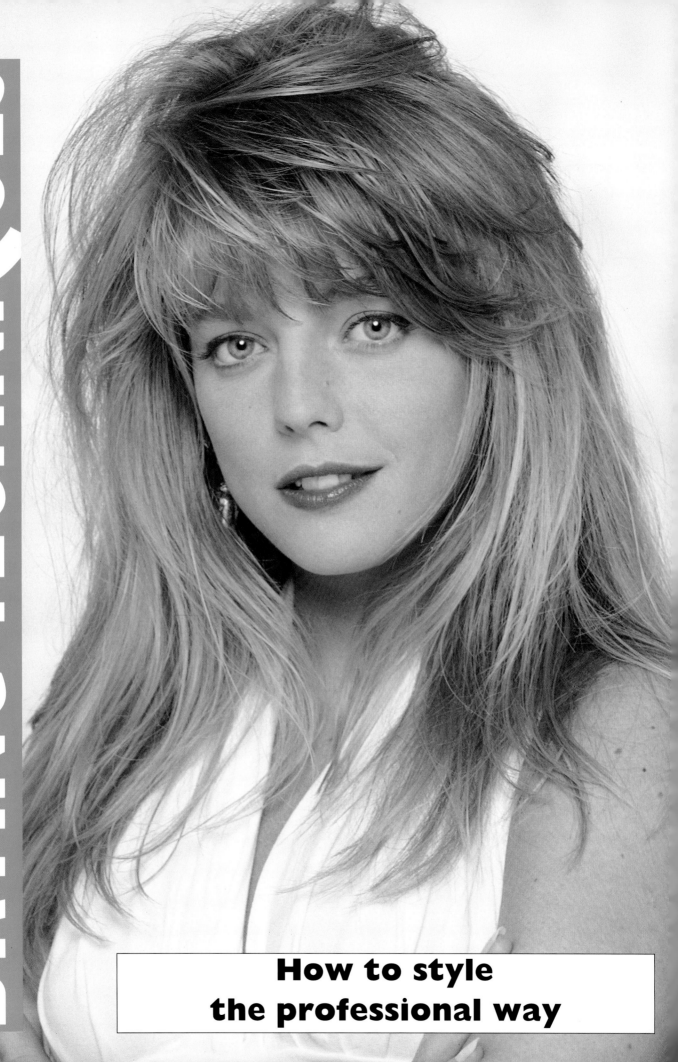

DRYING TECHNIQUES

**How to style
the professional way**

AIR DRYING

Constant blow-drying can be stressful to your hair leaving it dried out, dull and prone to split ends. Whenever possible pull the plug on your dryer and switch to natural, safe drying methods instead. You only need to use your fingers and – in an amazingly short time – any length of hair will be quite dry

Drying your hair with your hands is not as laborious as it sounds. Using just your fingers it's possible to scrunch, lift, comb, flick and twist all lengths of hair stylishly dry. And it really doesn't take very long. If you're doing it right short hair should be dry within five minutes and long hair within a quarter of an hour. The secret is to move your hands as quickly as possible through your hair to circulate the air which does all the drying for you.

MAKING WAVES

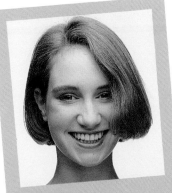

BEFORE
Capitalise on the curl in bob-length hair.

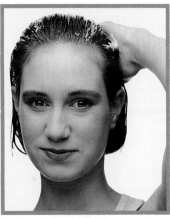

1 *Blot your hair with a towel so that it's no longer dripping wet. Comb it back and work a ping-pong ball sized blob of mousse through the roots.*

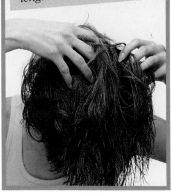

2 *Tip your head as far forwards as you can and repeatedly comb your fingers through from the roots down, moving as quickly as you can. Carry on until your hair looks dry but feels damp.*

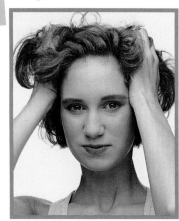

3 *Scrunch the ends of your hair towards your head with your hands, as if you are screwing up paper. This will encourage natural waves to form. Gently brush through.*

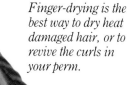

Tip

Finger-drying is the best way to dry heat damaged hair, or to revive the curls in your perm.

LONG HAIR

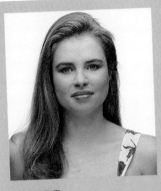

BEFORE
Finger-drying gives body and bounce to long hair, and emphasises natural curl.

1 ◀ After the final rinse, squeeze excess water off your hair with a towel so it's not dripping wet. Achieve lift by finger-drying the roots first. Flick your fingers rapidly through, close to your scalp, until it looks dry but feels damp.

2 ▶ Separate your hair into six sections and twist each one into a roll around your index finger. Secure with a hair grip. Leave in place for ten minutes.

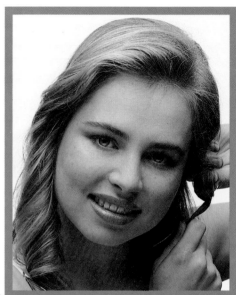

3 ◀ Remove grips and relax the rolls by combing with your fingers. Continue until you have the curl size that you want.

When drying your hair with your fingers, try to keep your hands as relaxed as possible. You'll get more movement, and avoid aching wrists!

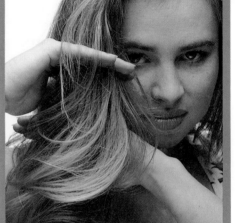

ANY QUESTIONS?

Q Can natural drying leave my long, curly perm too full to look good?

A Natural drying will always create volume through your hair, but you can control how much! Work on the ends for more fullness at the bottom than the top, concentrate on the roots for fullness throughout.

Q How do I know that my hair will suit natural drying techniques?

A The beauty of these techniques is that they suit all types of hair, and all lengths.

Of course, it's much quicker to dry short cropped hair than it is to dry a waist-length style.

Q I like to blow-dry my hair because it makes it shine. Can I get the same effect from natural drying?

A Shine is created when the cuticle on the hair shaft is made to lie flat so that light reflects off it. Blow-drying is only one way to achieve this look. For a really deep shine, condition your hair after shampooing, then dry it by rapidly brushing your fingers downwards through it.

Use gel on short styles and mousse on longer looks to help your hair hold its curls, but if your hair is already naturally curly then you can leave out this stage.

TOWEL TACTICS

● *Try not to rub your hair dry with a towel – you'll lift the cuticle layer on your hair leaving it vulnerable to damage. Squeezing and blotting is kinder.*

● *If you sleep on wet hair, put a towel on your pillow to absorb any wetness.*

● *The purpose of towel-drying is to stop your hair dripping water down your back and to speed up the drying process.*

● *Always move your hands away from the roots to keep the cuticle smooth, so that your hair will look shiny.*

AND SO TO BED . . .
You will not catch a cold, chill or flu from sleeping on wet hair. It's harmless!

SHORT HAIR

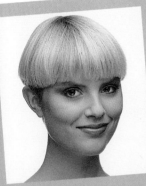

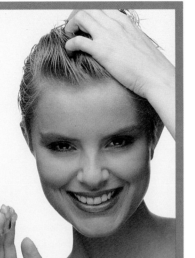

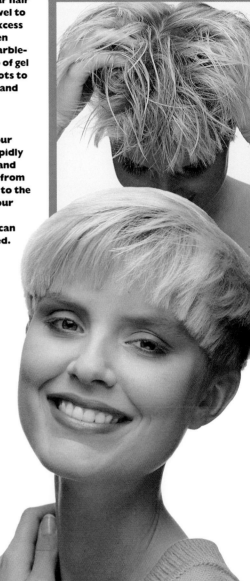

1 ◄ Blot your hair with a towel to remove excess water, then work a marble-sized blob of gel through the roots to help create lift and movement.

2 ► Run your fingers rapidly upwards and forwards from the roots to the ends of your hair. Do this as quickly as you can until it has dried.

BEFORE

Shorter hair dries quickly without help, but for a stylish look follow these three simple steps.

3 Bend your head forwards and spray hairspray into the roots. Stay put for one minute to give the spray time to dry and set your hair.

NATURAL DRYING ADDITIVES
A few extras to have at hand . . .
a towel
mousse or gel
a brush

SLEEP ON IT!

Don't lose precious beauty sleep because you have to dry your hair before going to bed. Just drop off wet . . . and wake up dry!

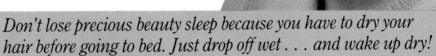

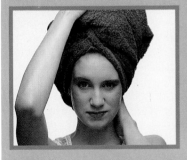

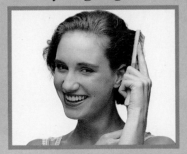

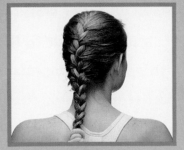

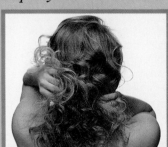

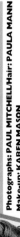

1 *You can dry hair of any length with the aid of a thick towel. Comb wet hair and wrap it up in a towel. Overnight it will retain the heat from your head, which will gently dry your hair.*

2 *In the morning, remove the towel and brush hair before styling.*

1 *Long hair can be curled overnight. Pat wet hair with a towel then plait it into a French plait, so that your hair is tight at the roots. Curl the ends under into the hair-tie to avoid straight tips.*

2 *In the morning your hair will be dry so gently release the plait and comb your fingers through to loosen the curl.*

Photographs: PAUL MITCHELL/Hair: PAULA MANN Make-up: KAREN MASON

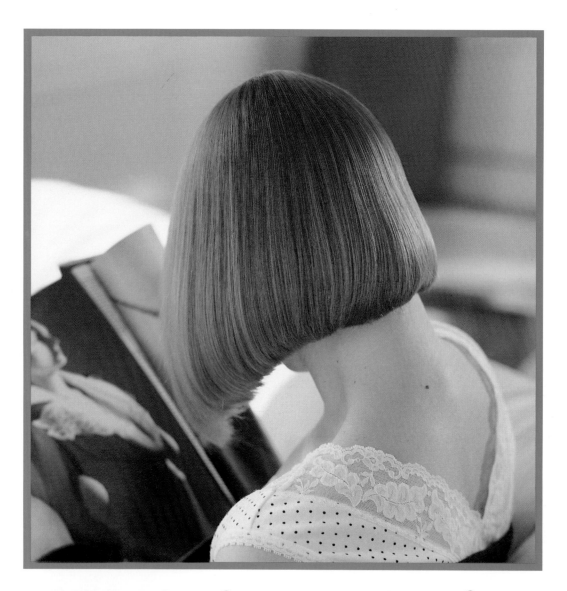

PUTTING ON THE SHINE

Photograph: LIZ McAULAY/Hair & Make-up: YA'NINA/Top: NEXT

Hair shine starts from within and your general health has a greater effect on the way it looks than you might think. Once a hair has emerged from the scalp it's effectively dead so whatever you eat can't affect the lengths – just the new growth. To ensure you're promoting healthy new hair eat a balanced diet that includes plenty of vitamin B complex, which is the most important one for shiny hair. It's no coincidence that many pet owners give it to their dogs for shiny coats!

Straight hair will always look more shiny than curly hair as its

Have you ever wondered how some people get their hair to look so wonderfully shiny? Is it completely natural or do they know something that you don't? Try these tips for no-fuss gloss

flat surface reflects light more easily. Similarly, darker hair will reflect more light than blonde hair. But don't despair if you're a curly blonde, because if you treat your hair carefully, always using conditioner after every wash and giving

your hair a regular deep conditioning treatment using oil, wax or cream, you should end up with glossy locks too.

For instant shine try rubbing a fingerful of wax down the lengths of freshly styled hair – it

works wonders on thick and coarse textures. But do take care to only use a little on very fine hair as it may become limp and lifeless.

Gloss sprays are perfect for all types of hair. They are simply a light oil in a spray form which coat the surface with a gentle mist without altering the shape or texture of your finished style.

Don't forget regular brushing too. While the brush goes through your hair it stimulates and distributes natural oils along the lengths and smoothes out all the tangles at the same time.

DRYING FOR SHINE

CHECK LIST
Styling mousse
Hairdryer
Flat-backed or
medium-sized
round brush
Hair clips
Extras: wax,
hairspray

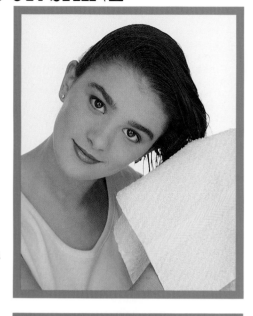

1 After washing, squeeze the excess water gently from your hair with a towel. Rub too vigorously and you'll get tangles.

2 For body and lasting hold squeeze a ball of mousse, about the size of a small egg, into the palm of one hand.

Forget the one about giving your hair 100 strokes a day. A good brushing helps to distribute natural oils, but too many can turn your scalp into an oil slick and damage the drier ends.

SHINE STRIPPERS
- Blow-drying and over-use of heated styling aids.
- Rough handling, especially when hair is wet.
- Insufficient rinsing after washing.
- Chemical treatments like perming and bleaching.
- Too much strong sun.
- Overloading hair with styling products.
- Dirty brushes and combs.

3 For maximum lift, work the mousse well into your hair, especially close to the roots. Add a little more if your hair is long.

Watchpoint

Try not to use too many sticky styling products like gels and waxes, especially if you live in a city. They attract the dirt, make your hair dull and encourage grease.

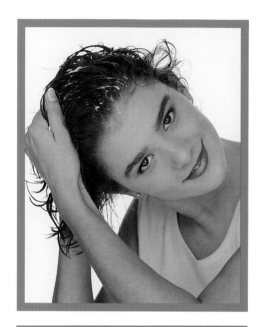

4 Rough-dry your hair first with a dryer. This cuts down the time it will take you to blow-dry. Stop when your hair feels slightly damp.

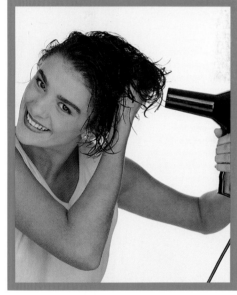

5 To blow-dry a smooth, sleek style use either a flat-backed or medium-sized round brush, with bristles that are fairly close together.

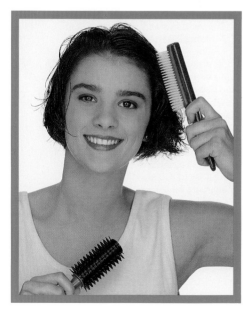

6 Brush all your hair over to one side and dry a bit more. This will give your hair extra lift as you are drying it away from the direction of growth. Once finished, repeat on the other side.

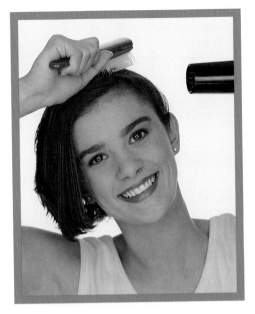

9 At the back of your head use the brush like a roller for the ends, curling the hair around it tightly while drying. For longer lasting hold leave the hair to cool for a couple of seconds before taking the brush out.

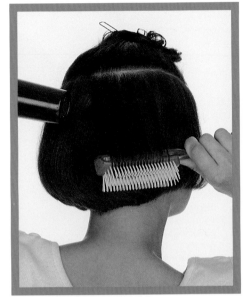

7 To make blow-drying easier it's best to work in sections, so make a parting all the way around your head and pin the top layer of hair up out of the way. By drying the underneath layer first you can give extra volume to your chosen style.

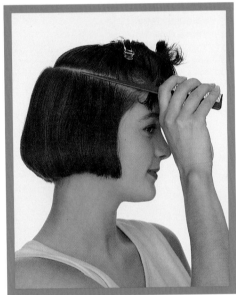

10 Once the bottom layer is dry, take down the rest of your hair and make a centre parting or a side parting according to your normal style.

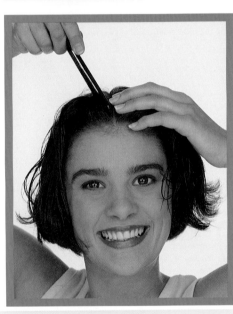

8 Start with the brush at the roots, then lift your hair while directing the dryer from the roots to the ends. Slowly move the brush down the length of hair holding it tightly all the time. Repeat this action all the way around using a small amount of hair at a time until it's all completely dry.

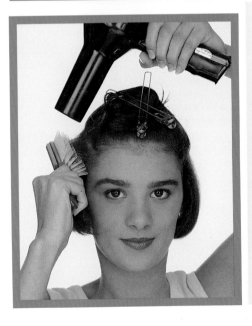

SHINE SAVERS

● Wash your hair in warm, not hot, water. Too hot water can damage the surface of the hair, dulling natural shine. Use cool water in the final rinses.

● Avoid using heated styling appliances every day as they tend to strip your hair of natural oils, leaving it dry.

● Use a heat styling lotion before blow-drying or a styling mousse which forms a protective barrier.

● Test your hairdryer on the back of your hand. If it's too hot for your skin to bear, it will be too hot for your hair, so switch to a lower heat setting.

● Split and frizzy ends will never look shiny, so remember to get them trimmed regularly.

● If you wash your hair every day, dilute your shampoo or choose one for frequent use. Coconut shampoo is good for shine.

● Always rinse your hair in fresh water after swimming in salt or chlorinated water.

● Check all your brushes and combs regularly for signs of wear and tear. Rough edges can damage your hair.

Photographs: ADRIAN BRADBURY/Hair: PENNY ATTWOOD/Make-up: YA'NINA

11 Start drying from the back leaving the front until last so you can match it up to the rest.

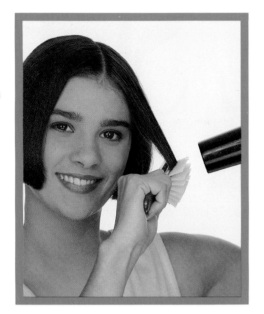

12 Your hair looks great! It's thicker and shinier than it has ever looked before, and with practice you'll find you can dry for shine in no time at all.

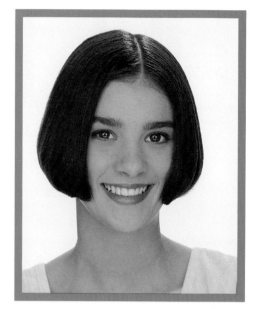

BEHIND THE SHEEN

A healthy lifestyle will go a long way towards getting your hair fighting fit!

● You may have read it 100 times before, but do try to stick to a balanced diet which includes plenty of fresh fruit and vegetables.

● Try to drink at least six glasses of water a day. Water helps to cleanse your system of impurities and makes your hair and skin look extra healthy.

● Try to take some regular exercise such as swimming or aerobics – a boost to your circulation will help your hair shine.

● If you've been a bit off-colour or feel that you are lacking certain vitamins in your diet, try taking supplements. Kelp (powdered seaweed) can be taken in a handy tablet form and is well known for its beneficial effect on hair.

● Vitamin B complex is another hair shine goodie. This can be found in yeast extract, eggs, liver and wholegrains, or you can take it as a supplement in tablet form.

● While you're watching TV or as part of your shampoo routine, give your scalp a soothing massage. This helps to stimulate blood circulation and encourages healthy new hair growth.

● Cut down on sugary foods as they destroy vitamin B – as well as your teeth!

● All that fresh air may be good for you but make sure your hair's protected from the drying effects of sun and wind when you're out and about.

● Central heating will dry your hair and skin out – but if you can't live without it, treat yourself to a humidifier to put the moisture back into the air.

FINISHING OFF

Try these professional tricks for a photo finish.

● Warm and soften a fingerful of hair wax using a hairdryer and smooth over your hair for the ultimate shine.

● Spritz a little finishing spray onto a comb and run it through your hair to prevent static.

● Add a drop of rosemary oil to your brush to stop tangles forming and eliminate static.

● Get instant gloss with a few drops of spray-on shine. Keep it light though, or you could end up looking like your hair needs a wash.

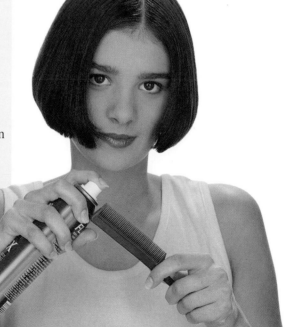

IN A SLEEK CONDITION

If your hair lacks shine make sure you:

● Always use a conditioner.

● Treat your hair once a week to a deep conditioning treatment. Use a cream or wax formula and leave on for 30 minutes.

● Try a hot oil treatment if your hair is out of condition or your scalp dry. Warm a tablespoon of vegetable oil and massage into your hair. Wrap in cling film and leave on as long as possible before shampooing out.

● Make your own natural conditioner from mashed avocado, raw egg, natural yoghurt or home made mayonnaise. Leave on your hair for ½ hour and rinse well.

● Pour ½ a cup of cider vinegar over your hair as a finishing rinse after shampooing for sleek hair.

● If you're blonde, squeeze a lemon over your hair instead of conditioner – it'll pick up highlights as well as shine.

● Put your conditioner on while you're in the bath – the steam will make the treatment penetrate into your hair.

DO THE SCRUN

Scrunch-drying your hair is as easy as crumpling a piece of paper in your hand. Here's how to add a truly professional finish to short, medium and long styles

Ever wished you could make your hair look as good at home as it does when you leave the salon? Well, there's one technique popular with hairdressers that's *really* easy to copy – it's called scrunch-drying and it's a great way of giving extra volume and bounce to your hair.

Scrunching works best on layered hair, but you can use the technique on one-length hair that isn't too long (chin to shoulder length is best), as well as short, or naturally curly hair. All you need is some styling mousse and a blow dryer. If your hair's short, or cut in a bob, your usual

SCRUNCHING A BOB

Use the scrunching technique on shoulder-length hair, and Bob's your uncle – you'll have a style that's full of body and bounce.

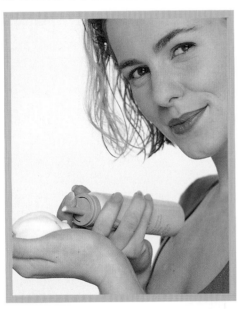

1 Start with freshly washed, towel-dried hair. Squirt an egg-sized blob of styling mousse into one hand. Choose firm hold mousse for fine/normal hair; normal hold for thick/coarse hair.

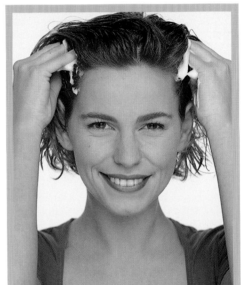

2 Work about half the mousse into the roots on one side of your hair. Use the rest on the other side. Use both hands to make sure you spread it right down to the ends.

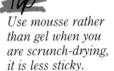
Tip
Use mousse rather than gel when you are scrunch-drying, it is less sticky.

4 On a bob, scrunch from halfway down the length of the hair to the ends by literally screwing up a handful of hair in one hand. Hold for a count of five, aiming your hairdryer at the gaps between your fingers. Keep on scrunching all around your head.

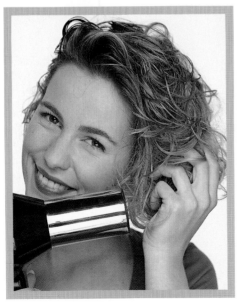

5 For maximum volume tip your head forwards and blow-dry the underneath of your hair using your fingers to lift and squeeze the roots. The finished effect should be tousled, soft and it should not look too neat.

Tip
If the heat is too much for your fingers to bear, then it's too hot for your hair to handle!

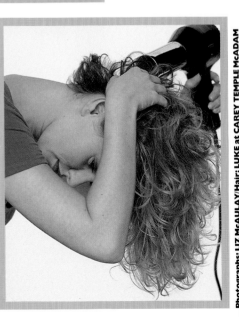

Photographs: LIZ McAULAY/Hair: LUKE at CAREY TEMPLE McADAM

CH!

dryer will do, if it's long or curly, adding a diffuser attachment to the dryer will help.

All you have to do is work the mousse into your roots and scrunch your hair by screwing up handfuls of hair. Follow this up with a bit of clever blow-drying for a fantastic carefree style.

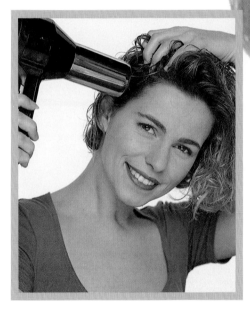

3 Using your hairdryer on a medium heat, rough dry until your hair is only slightly damp. Use your fingers to lift the hair at the roots, pushing it back around your hairline to give lots of face-framing volume.

6 When the finished effect looks exactly as you want it, set the style with a light mist of hairspray.

Salon secrets

For a scrunch that lasts, lift your hair and aim hairspray straight at the roots.

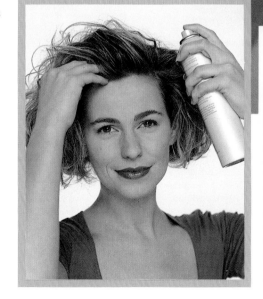

ANY QUESTIONS?

Q How do I know if my hair will suit scrunching?

A Scrunching suits just about any type of hair that has a wave. As long as your hair isn't too fine or completely shorn it should look great.

Q How long will the effects of scrunching last on my hair?

A Your hair should stay looking good all day. If you want it to last longer you can add a dot of wax. Rub this between the palms of both hands for even coverage.

Q Will scrunching do any damage?

A No. But if your hair is very dry, or over coloured, the heat from the hairdryer might. So if you're worried, dry your hair naturally, and then scrunch. Use a hairdryer on a low setting, and buy a special diffuser attachment to spread the heat.

TWICE AS NICE

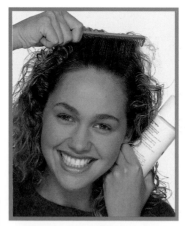

1 Wash and towel-dry your hair. Comb a grapefruit-sized blob of mousse or a walnut-sized blob of gel evenly through your hair.

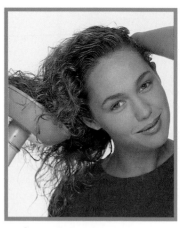

2 Scrunch-dry the ends by grabbing handfuls of hair and gently lifting them up as you direct the air from the diffuser onto them. Don't dry the front yet.

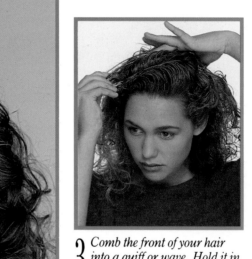

3 Comb the front of your hair into a quiff or wave. Hold it in place with a section clip. Make another two waves – behind the front one – and clip in place.

Tip

Add bags of body to your hair by tipping your head forwards and scrunch-drying the back.

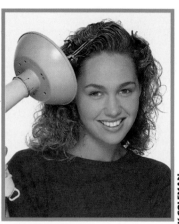

4 Point the hairdryer with diffuser attachment at the waves you have just made and dry them thoroughly. Leave your hair to cool.

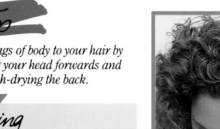

5 Remove the clips carefully without disturbing the waves. Fluff up the ends of your hair using your fingers. Tip your head forwards and shake it to add body.

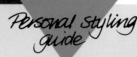

Personal styling guide

◆ easy

🕐 quick to style

✳ **Works best on** one-length or layered wavy hair or any type of hair that scrunches easily.

☑ **You need:**
comb
mousse or gel
hairdryer with diffuser attachment
section clips

Photographs: NICK COLE/Hair/Make-up: KAREN PURVIS/Top: NICK COLEMAN

SCRUNCHING SHORT HAIR

Short hair can benefit from a bit of bounce. Dry from the roots for extra lift.

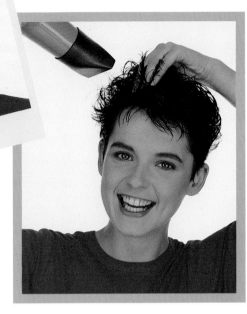

BEFORE:
a short, straight cut.

1 ◄ Work a small blob of mousse through damp hair. Grasp your hair firmly by the roots and lift as you dry. Use a hairdryer with a nozzle attachment.

2 ► Keep drying the top layers until they are completely dry, and there you have it – a sophisticated style with body and lift.

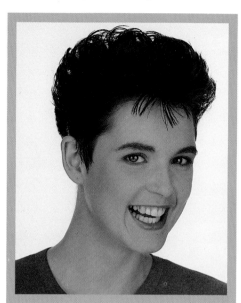

HOT AIR DIFFUSER

This bowl-shaped hairdryer attachment is invaluable for drying curls without frizz. It's also gentler on your hair than a straightforward hairdryer. Some dryers are sold with a diffuser, but if you buy one separately, make sure it fits the dryer you've got at home!

SCRUNCHING CURLS

Scrunch-drying is not just for making waves, it's also a way of drying natural curls and perms.

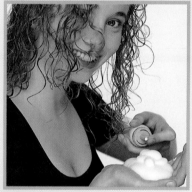

1 Use a blob of styling mousse on your hair. Firm hold is ideal for fine/normal hair, and normal hold for thick, permed hair.

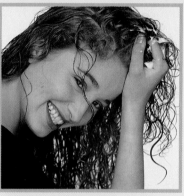

2 Work half the mousse well into the roots, then use your fingers to work the rest of the mousse through to the ends.

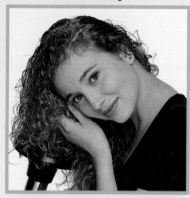

3 Bend your head forwards and hold the hairdryer below your hair, so it's pointing upwards.

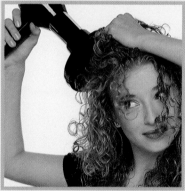

4 Scrunch up handfuls of hair while you're drying it. To dry the top sections of hair, hold the dryer a couple of inches above your hair. Scrunch up handfuls until you have a headful of soft curls.

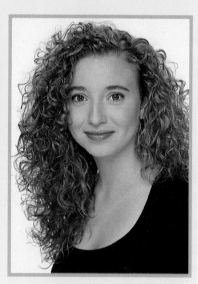

Photographs: ADRIAN BRADBURY/Black top: PINEAPPLE

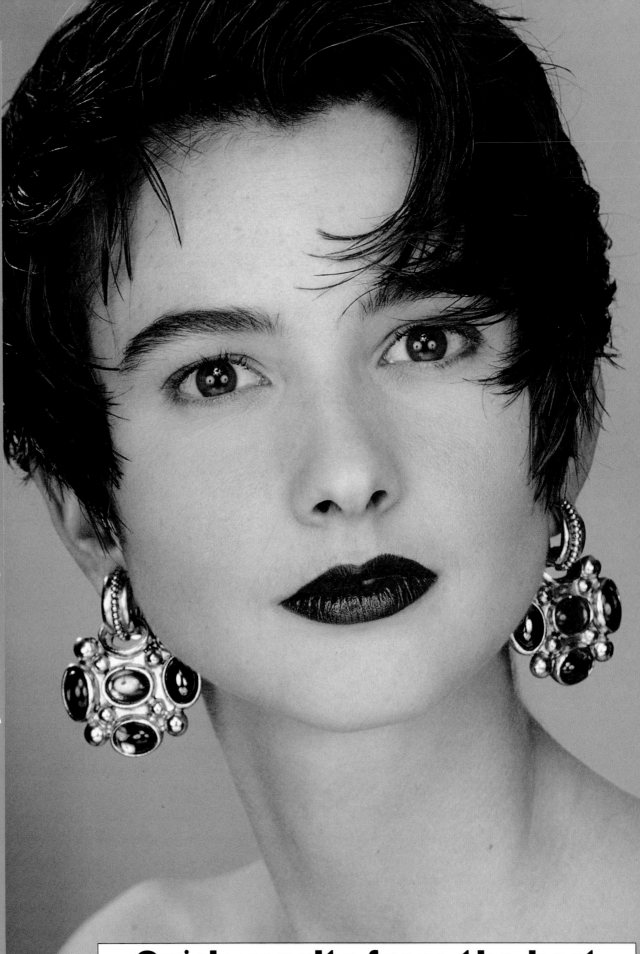

MOUSSE, GEL, WAX & SPRAY

Quick results from the best products for you

SUPER MOUSSE

Mousse makes light work of hair styling – for natural body and bounce, you'll find it's all in the can!

These days if you want body, shape and manageability for your hair then you need look no further than a can of mousse. It's actually a setting agent in foam form. The foam helps spread it through your hair, then dissolves, leaving a fine coating of resins to help you shape your hair. Canned mousse also contains a chemical propellant which turns it from liquid to foam when it leaves the container. Help mix them into a firm foam with a quick shake before use. The latest mousses come in squeezy plastic bottles and are propellant-free. They use an air-pump which makes a light and fluffy mousse – and should not be shaken before use.

GET IT RIGHT!

For best results, always use the right amount of mousse – too little and the style will flop, too much and you'll make it dull and sticky.
- On short hair use an egg-sized blob of mousse.
- On medium-length, short Afro or permed hair, use an orange-sized blob.
- On long Afro, permed and very long straight hair, use a grape-fruit-sized blob.

Never put mousse straight on to your hair. Rub a small blob over your palms, then spread it through your hair. If you're using a big blob, scoop up a manageable amount and work into hair section by section.

HEATWAVE

Mousse doesn't just work when hair's wet – it can give dry hair a whole new look, too.

WHICH ONE TO CHOOSE

Mousse comes in several different strengths – choose one to suit your hair and styling needs.
NORMAL HOLD – for daily use on normal hair.
EXTRA/SUPER HOLD – contains an extra bonding agent. Use it for elaborate styles or on very fine or flyaway hair.
CONDITIONING MOUSSE – leaves a sheen on your hair. Good choice if you blow-dry as the extra conditioners help protect your hair from the heat, but the conditioner may weaken the hold.

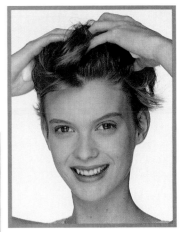

1 *Massage an egg-sized blob of mousse thoroughly into your roots, pushing your hair back from your forehead as you go.*

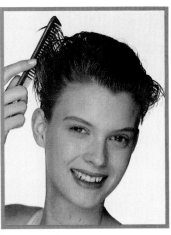

2 *Comb through to spread the mousse from the roots to the ends and to encourage your hair to lie flat and smooth.*

Photographs: IAN HOOTON/Hair: PENNY ATTWOOD/Make-up: LIZZIE COURT/Vest: KNICKERBOX Silk jacket: FRENCH CONNECTION/Earrings: NEC;CESSORY

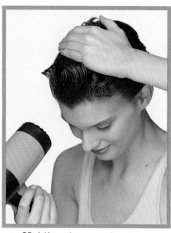

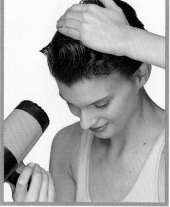

3 With clean palms, push the top section of your hair forwards into a gentle wave so that the hairline roots are lifted away from your forehead.

4 Holding the wave in place, blow-dry on a high setting for two to three minutes to dry the mousse and set your hair.

FRIZZ-FREE VOLUME

Mousse keeps curls under control when blow-drying.

Afro and permed hair is very porous so it will absorb mousse quickly. Don't judge by looks alone. Feel your hair – it should be slightly sticky, but not tacky.

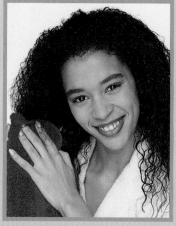

1 Towel-dry wet hair to remove excess water. Blot rather than rub it, which can roughen the surface and cause tangles.

Tip

Don't worry if your hair's not squeaky clean, a little natural oil will give the style more staying power.

Tip

Concentrated heat can harm your hair, so it's much safer to move the dryer away for a few moments to 'rest' in between hot blasts.

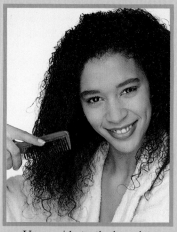

4 Use a wide-toothed comb to spread the mousse evenly down the length of your hair.

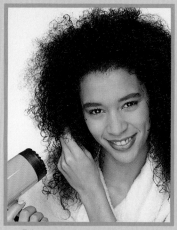

5 Blow-dry your hair using your fingers to shape and separate the curls. If the ends are still frizzy once it's dry rub in a marble-sized blob of mousse.

SCRUNCH BUNCH

If your hair's dry or damaged, it's kinder to wave it by hand!

If your hair is thick, it may still be damp after an hour's wrapping, so re-wrap it in a warmed dry towel to speed up the drying.

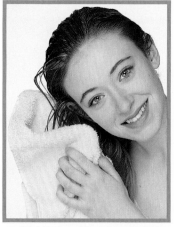

1 Lightly towel-dry your hair to remove excess water. Blot away as much as you can to shorten the towel-wrap drying time later.

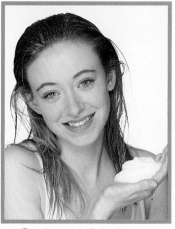

2 Comb your hair back to get rid of any tangles. Squirt an orange-sized blob of mousse into one hand.

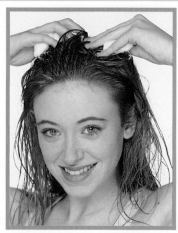

3 Start to work the mousse through your hair by gently massaging it into the roots.

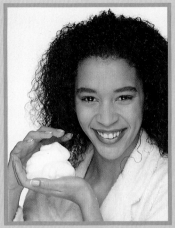

2 Squirt a grapefruit-sized blob of mousse into one hand. You'll need less if your hair is shorter than in our picture.

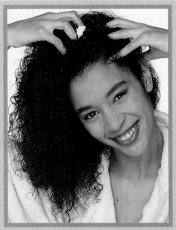

3 Dip your fingers in the mousse to give lots of small blobs. Massage these into the roots.

MOUSSE MIX

Polish up your act! Mix wax with mousse for super shine and extra sleek control.

Rubbing wax thoroughly in your palms will warm and melt it slightly so it's much easier to use. If it's not warmed the wax may form thick clumps in your hair when you work it through.

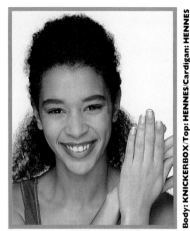

1 Take a thumbnail-sized blob of wax and rub it between your palms until very smooth.

Body: KNICKERBOX/Top: HENNES/Cardigan: HENNES

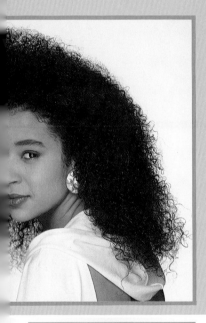

QUICK TIPS

● Mousses do vary – some are stickier than others, so you should use a little less; others are watery and you may need more than usual. To test a new mousse squirt a blob on to one hand, rub your palms together, then slowly pull them apart to see whether they feel tacky or watery.

● Work mousse into your hair quickly so it doesn't dry on your hands.

● Don't forget to spread the mousse on your back hair and along your hairline.

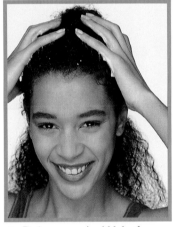

2 Rub an egg-sized blob of mousse into your waxed palms. Smooth it over your hair. 'Comb' moussed fingers through the ends to separate curls.

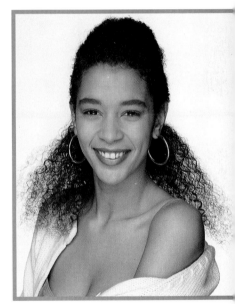

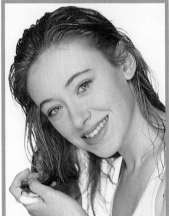

4 Work it through the ends of your hair by scrunching with moussed palms. This will encourage loose waves to form.

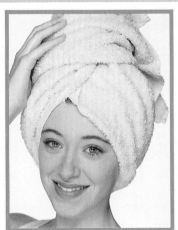

5 Take a warmed dry towel and wrap it around your head. Leave your hair to dry for about an hour.

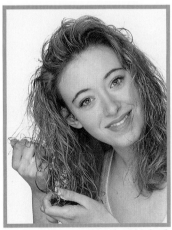

6 Smooth a marble-sized blob of mousse over your fingers and give the dried curls a final scrunch into shape.

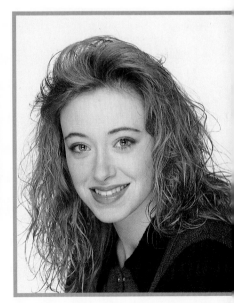

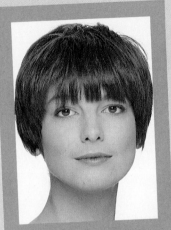

BEFORE
Start with freshly-washed, towel-dried hair.

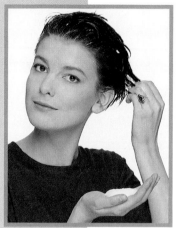

1 *Smooth an egg-sized blob of mousse through your hair from the roots to the ends.*

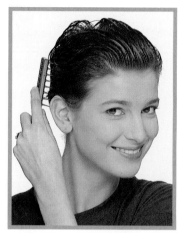

2 *Brush your hair through using a vent brush to help spread the mousse evenly.*

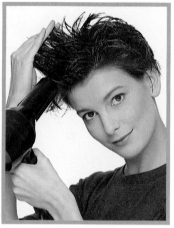

3 *Dry using your fingers to lift hair up and away from your head. Make sure you dry the roots first to give maximum lift.*

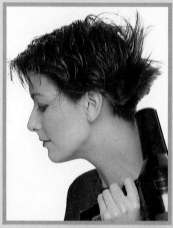

4 *Tip your head forwards slightly and dry the back section, keeping the hairdryer pointing upwards to give root lift.*

Cropped hair can reach the height of fashion with this spiky style. Just arm yourself with mousse and a hairdryer and go all out for the high life

HAIR RAISER

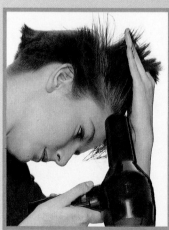

5 *Continue to dry the front and side sections in the same way, remembering to lift the hair with your fingers as you go.*

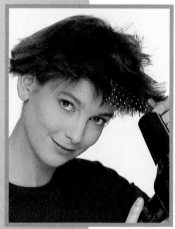

6 *Soften the fringe by putting the flat side of the vent brush against your forehead and gently drying the hair over it.*

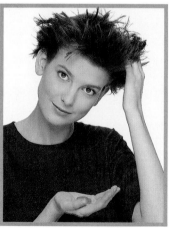

7 *Finish by working a marble-sized blob of gel through the hair to give shine and hold.*

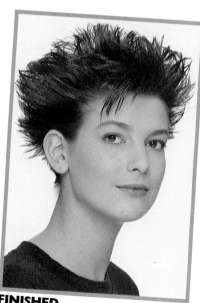

FINISHED

Hair gel is good news for short styles, his and yours, to give lift, shape and long-lasting hold. Here's how to transform two basic cuts with just one tube of sticky stuff!

GEL KNOW HOW

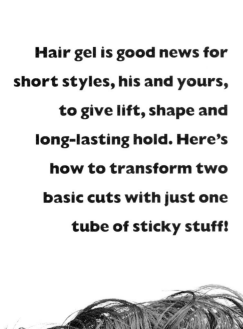
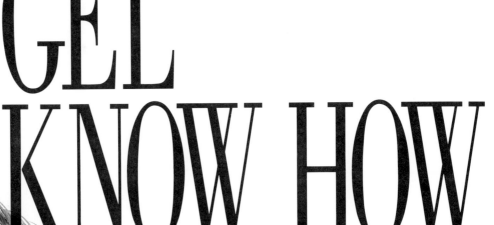

If you like to change your hairstyle as often as your clothes, then hair gel is for you! Just a handful of gel can sculpt, wave or set your hair into a style that will last from dawn until dusk. With a little imagination you can give a simple short cut a different look for every day of the week, according to your outfit or mood.

Gel is available in lots of different colours, none of which makes any difference to the end result. What does make a difference is the amount of gel that you put on – too little and your style won't stay, too much and you'll look as if you haven't washed your hair for a fortnight!

Work in gel sparingly and remember that you can always add more, but you can't take it away without washing your hair again.

WHAT'S WHAT

All gel formulations can be used on towel-dried or dry hair.

Normal hold: for softer, overall hold. Use to emphasise a fringe or add texture to a layered cut.

Extra hold: for high hair and spiky styles. The best formulation for holding fine hair in place.

Wet-look: for slicked back, glossy styles. Remains pliable rather than setting rock hard.

GEL FOR THE GIRLS

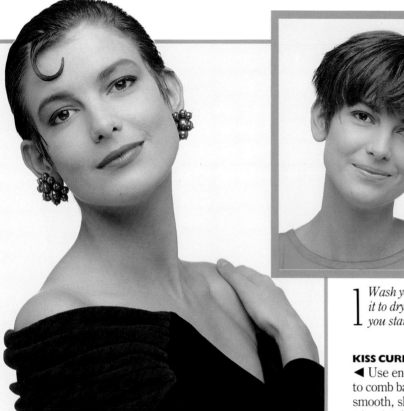

Dress: MISS SELFRIDGE/Earrings: HENNES

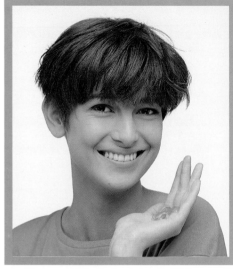

1 *Wash your hair and allow it to dry thoroughly before you start. Comb through.*

2 *Squeeze a marble-sized blob of gel into the palm of one hand. Rub your palms together to spread the gel.*

KISS CURL GIRL

◄ Use enough gel to enable you to comb back your hair into a smooth, sleek finish. Section a triangle of hair on the front hairline, gel it and hold in a curl shape with your fingers until it dries. Avoid sticking the curl to your forehead and put on your make-up first so that you don't have to disturb your work of art!

UPTOWN GIRL

► Look chic by sculpting and smoothing the front section of your hair up and over, using your fingers and palms to secure the shape while the gel dries. Finish by stroking and smoothing back the sides of your hair.

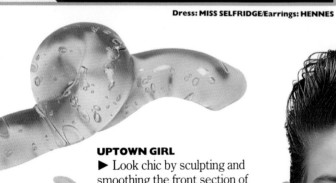

If you're a regular gel user and your hair starts to look a little dull, switch to using an anti build-up shampoo until the shine returns.

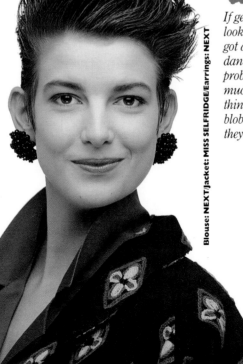

Blouse: NEXT/Jacket: MISS SELFRIDGE/Earrings: NEXT

Tip

If gel leaves you looking as if you've got a bad attack of dandruff, you're probably using too much. Use only a thin film, rather than blobs which flake as they dry.

NEW WAVE

► For a more heavily sculptured look you will need to put on slightly more gel and comb it through. Slide your palm up and back across the side of your head and hold the wave in place with your hands until the gel has dried. Smooth back the sides, adding a touch more gel to tame any stray hairs.

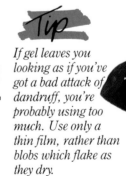

SOFT & GENTLE

▼ Use your fingers to flick your hair in all directions to achieve lift and volume. Now bring it all forwards from the back of your head into a full fringe. By adding a little more gel to some sections you can create different textures and movement.

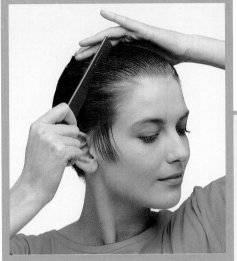

3 *Put it on the roots of your hair first and then smooth it down to the ends with your fingers for an even coating.*

4 *A quick flick through with a comb and you're ready to start styling.*

If you've used a little gel to add texture and lift, this should disappear with a good brushing. If you've used a lot or a wet-look formulation you'll have to shampoo.

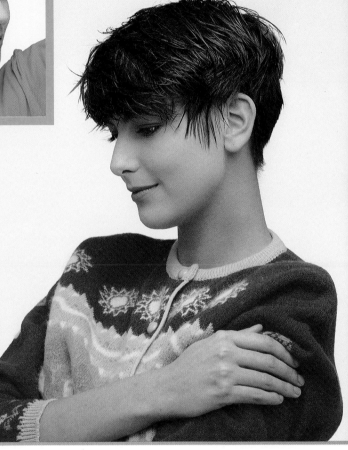

Cardigan: BENETTON

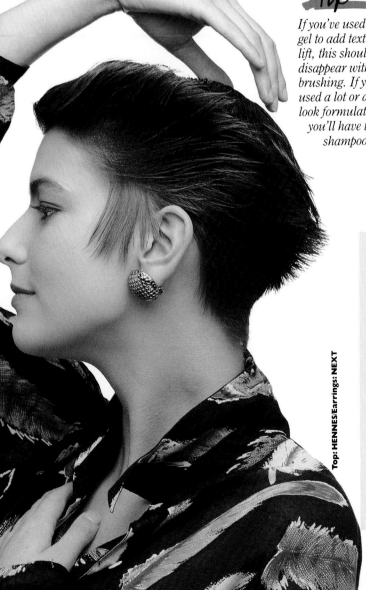

Top: HENNES/Earrings: NEXT

GEL TRICKS

AFRO
Beat the frizzies by applying extra hold gel with your fingers, just to the ends, and pulling small strands of hair straight.

PLAITS
Run a little gel along a finished plait to smooth down stray hairs and create a sleek look.

VOLUME
Rub into the roots while your hair is still damp then finger-dry, directing the heat from the hair-dryer under rather than on top of your hair to give some lift.

SLEEK
To cover up hair that's looking less than lovely, or to hide growing out layers, put gel on dry hair and comb into place. You'll need one marble-sized blob upto shoulder length and two blobs if it is any longer.

BOBS
Smooth gel lightly over the surface of any one-length style, such as a bob, instead of hairspray.

CURLS
Use a wet-look gel to smooth over permed or naturally curly hair to add a glossy shine and to separate the curls.

GEL FOR THE BOYS

Shirt and tie: NEXT/Jacket: BLAZER

CITY SLICKER
◀ For a sleek finish apply another small blob of gel and comb through. Part your hair with a comb and shape the front section into an S-shaped wave. Comb the sides to lie smooth and flat about your ears.

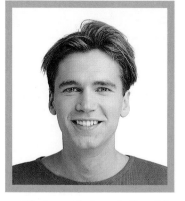

1 Wash your hair and allow it to dry thoroughly before you start. Comb it through.

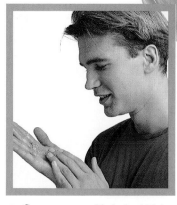

2 Squeeze a marbled-sized blob of gel into the palm of one hand and rub palms together.

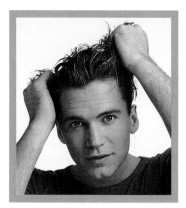

3 Work the gel into your hair from the roots right to the ends with your fingertips.

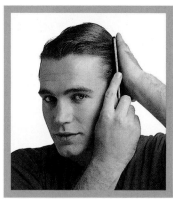

4 Comb through lightly to get an even spread, and now it's time to get creative!

Photographs: PAUL MITCHELL/Hair & make-up: CHASE ASTON

Shirt: KATHERINE HAMNETT

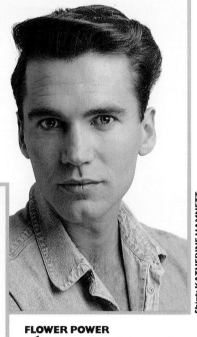

FLOWER POWER
◀ Lift your front hair up and over and hold in place with your hands until the gel dries. Using your palms, smooth back the sides and back of your hair. Tame strays hairs with a little extra gel.

Shirt: HENNES

STYLE KING
▶ Lift the front section of hair up and over using your hands and hold in position until the gel dries. Pay special attention to smoothing the sides to create a contrast with the lifted top piece. To achieve the cross-over look, smooth the sides to meet at the back.

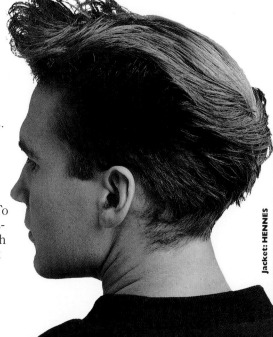

Jacket: HENNES

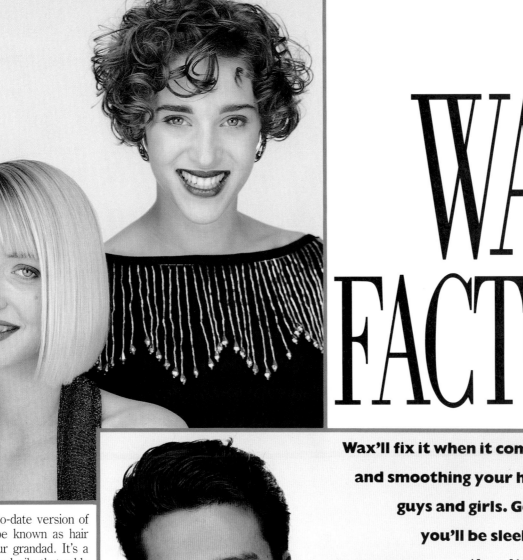

Photographs: ADRIAN BRADBURY/Hair: MIA/Make-up: TRACEY LERMAN/Man's waistcoat and shirt: NEXT/Red jacket: MONSOON/Dresses: MISS SELFRIDGE/Earrings: HARVEY NICHOLS

WAX FACTOR

Wax'll fix it when it comes to shaping and smoothing your hair — for both guys and girls. Get it right and you'll be sleeks ahead with the ultimate in shine

Wax is the up-to-date version of what used to be known as hair dressing by your grandad. It's a mix of waxes and oils that adds softness, body and shine to your hair without leaving it greasy.

Hair wax is water resistant so you can't use it on wet hair. It can also be fairly difficult to wash out unless it's a water-soluble wax so check the label before you buy. However, it works wonders on all types of freshly dried hair as it's strong enough to structure curls, add root lift and smooth for a perfect, professional finish.

If you use mousse, gel or setting lotion put wax on styled and dried hair to stop it looking dull. And you can restore the shine to hair that has lost its lustre thanks to perming or colouring with – you guessed! – wax.

If you want to get rid of a non-water soluble wax put a little shampoo on dry hair, massage well then wash as usual.

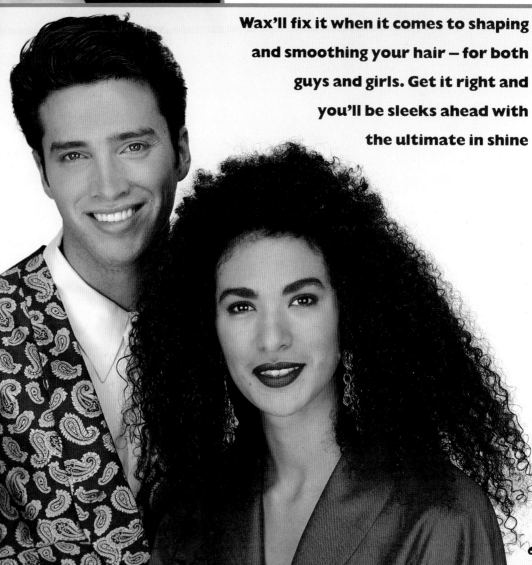

61

GET IT ON

The way you put wax on your hair makes all the difference when you're after a stylish, non-greasy effect.

Tip

Keep the lid tightly closed if you don't want a pot of wax to harden.

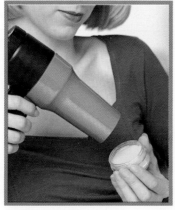

1 *If the wax is too solid, gently warm it with a hairdryer on a cool setting until the surface is slightly runny.*

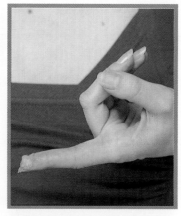

2 *Start with just a thumbnail-sized blob. You can always add more if you need to.*

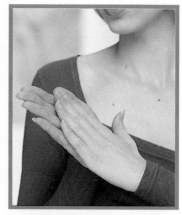

3 *Always spread the wax over your hands first. This warms the wax and makes it easier to smooth evenly over your hair.*

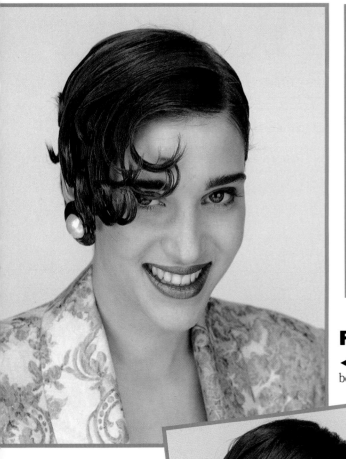

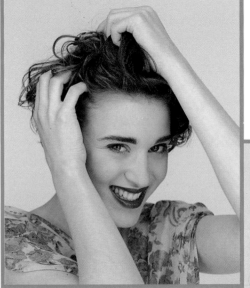

Watchpoint

Only use wax on really clean hair as it will make hair greasy if there's any excess natural oils.

FINGER CURLS

◄ Wax coated hair can quickly and easily be moulded into face framing curls. Just smooth some wax through the hair then take 12 mm/½ in sections and twist into individual curls with your fingers. Set with a hairdryer on a cool setting, then pull the curls forwards and arrange them to frame your face.

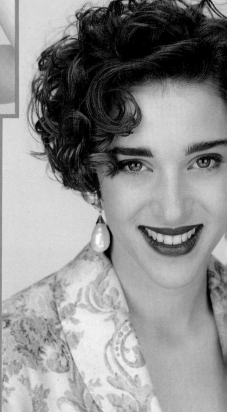

Watchpoint

If you're prone to oily skin don't bring waxed hair forwards on to your face.

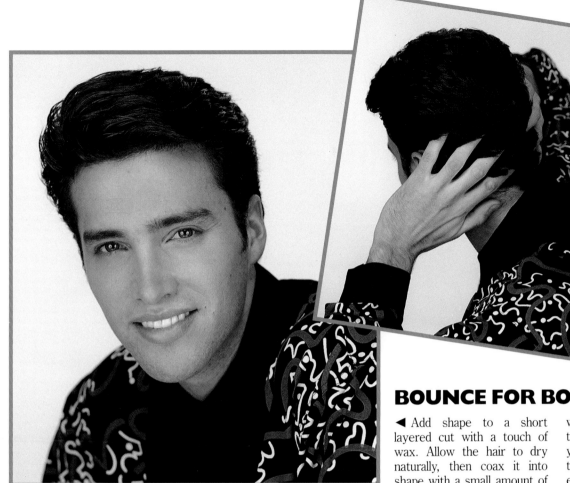

Watchpoint

Don't sleep on it! When you use wax make sure that you shampoo your hair before you hit the pillow or you'll suffer the greasy consequences in the morning!

BOUNCE FOR BOYS

◀ Add shape to a short layered cut with a touch of wax. Allow the hair to dry naturally, then coax it into shape with a small amount of wax paying particular attention to the front and sides. Smooth your hands through from roots to ends so that the finished effect doesn't look too solid.

MAKING WAVES

▶ Use a little more wax and add some rippling waves. Start at the front hairline and run wax back through your hair. Push the top section forwards into a wave with one hand, and secure with three long clips. Fix the waves in place with a hairdryer on a gentle heat setting.

Tip

Banish a wispy hairline with just a little wax when you've finished creating a neat upswept style.

CURL UP

◀ Wax adds definition and texture to naturally curly and permed hair. Lightly massage the wax through short hair with lots of curls, starting at the roots. Use your fingers to lift the front section to flatter your face, then gently tease the curls into shape. The result is curls with added body and texture as well as long lasting hold.

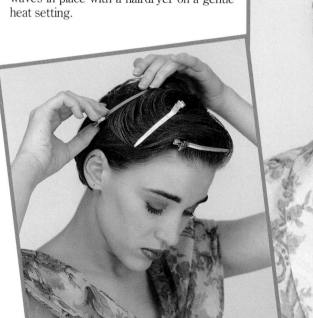

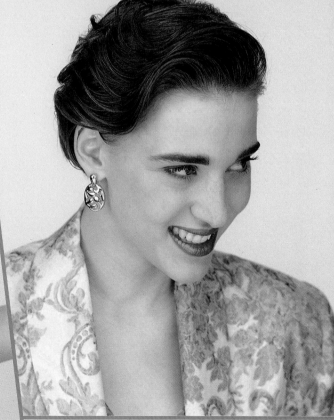

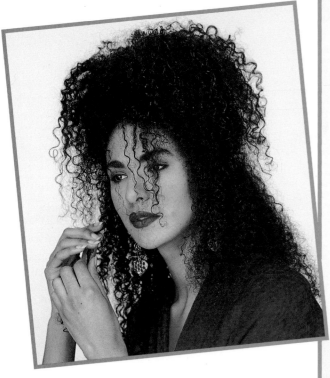

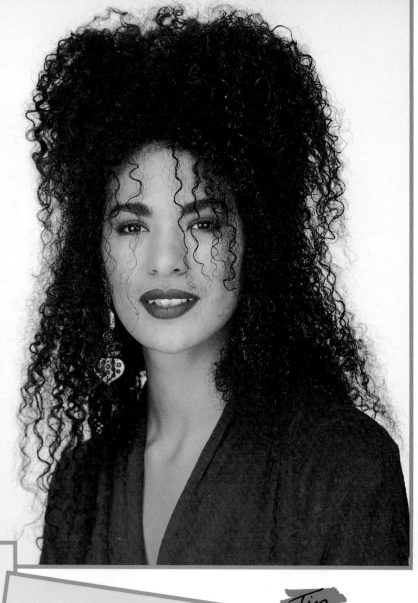

FRIZZ FREE

▶ Wax is Afro hair's best friend, helping to separate the curls, add shine and beat the frizzies. Spread wax evenly through your hair, from roots to ends. Working in small sections literally 'squeeze' the wax into your hair until you've eliminated frizziness and defined the curls.

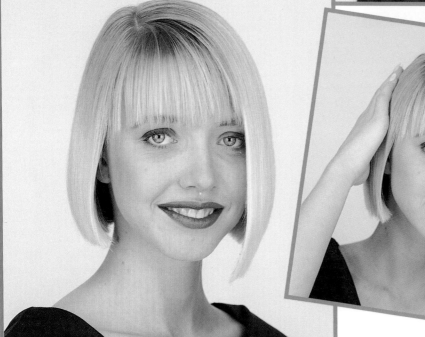

Wax smoothes down the surface of the hair and helps prevent static electricity that makes it frizz.

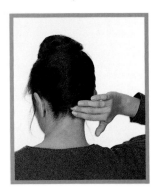

SMOOTH OPERATOR

◀ Use wax to smooth down stray hairs on a sleek style and add a healthy shine. Blow-dry your hair in the usual way, then run wax-coated hands over the surface. Use the remaining wax on your hands to lightly separate the fringe, and you'll have a glossy look that's ultra-sophisticated. It's also a great way to give damaged hair gloss too.

HOLDING POWER

Hairspray used to be stiff stuff, but it now gives a much more natural look. And it's versatile – use it to set your style, hold it, add body or control flyaway ends

Hairsprays are still the best-selling hair styling product – and most fall into one of two main categories – traditional 'holding' sprays which fix hair, or the newer styling sprays. Some, however, cleverly combine both actions.

Holding hairsprays come in either aerosols or pump action sprays. Most aerosols are now free of CFCs – the chemicals that threaten the ozone layer. Almost all styling sprays come in pump action packs.

Aerosols discharge a very fine mist, which dries quickly. Pump action hairsprays tend to come out quite wet, so need a couple of seconds in which to dry. These can be too heavy for fine hair.

Holding sprays are available in various strengths: normal/natural, extra firm, or mega-hold. The stronger the hold, the more alcohol and resins in the spray.

The closer you hold the nozzle to your head, the wetter the spray will be and the firmer the hold it will give. Hold aerosols at least 15 cm/6 in away.

ON THE SHELF

Confused by all the choices in the shops? Our guide will help you:

AEROSOL HAIRSPRAY Use to give support to your style, and as finishing spray. It's suitable for all hair types, especially fine or floppy hair.

CONDITIONING HAIRSPRAY Acts like hairspray, but contains conditioners, which make it good for chemically-treated and dry hair. It also adds shine.

STYLING SPRAY Usually comes in a pump action pack and can be used on damp hair to shape and on dry hair to hold. Many also contain conditioners. It's good for all hair types. Also known as styling spritz, sculpting mist, fixing spray or spray fix.

VOLUMISING SPRAY Unlike most sprays, which just coat the outside of the hair shaft, this type penetrates the follicle to give inner strength. Special resins coat each strand to thicken hair. It also styles either dry or damp hair. It's good for all hair types, especially fine, flyaway hair needing body.

SPRAY-ON SHINE This is similar to a conditioning hairspray and will add lustre to your finished look. Some brands combine spray-on shine with holding power.

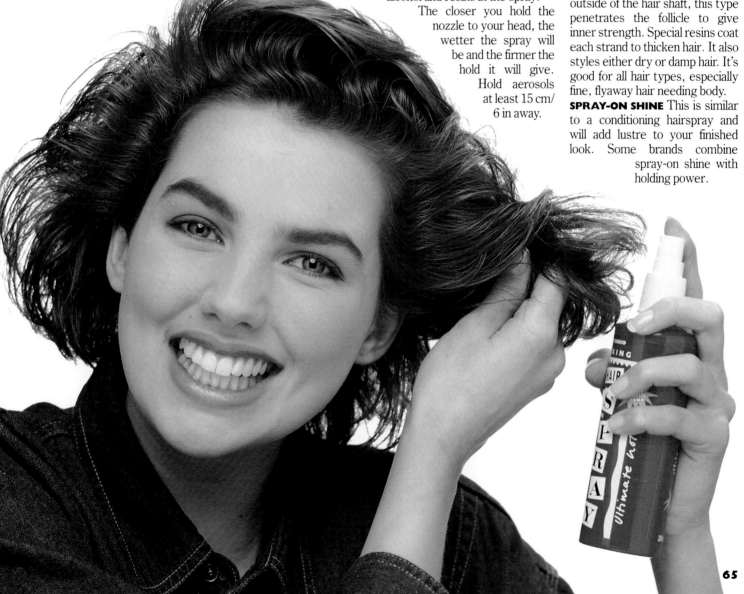

SLEEK IS CHIC

For a chic chignon, plait or French pleat, use spray-on shine to give hair a sleek finish and help fight static.

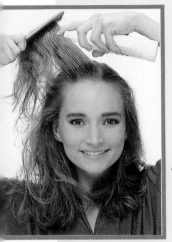

1 Comb holding spray through clean, dry hair before you start.

For a smooth finish, make the hair quite wet with spray before you style it.

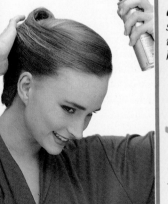

2 When you've put your hair up as you want it, use a spray-on shine to give it gloss. This will also help to hold hair.

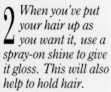

Watchpoint

Touch-up with spray from a distance – if the hair gets too wet strands will separate.

3 A good squirt of spray round the hairline will stop stray hairs from escaping and spoiling the sleek line.

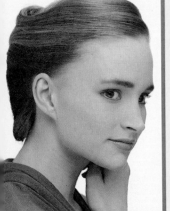

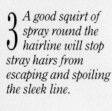

As you spray, smooth hair with your free hand to keep straggly strands in place.

FAST FORWARD

To achieve a textured look on short hair, use a volumising spray.

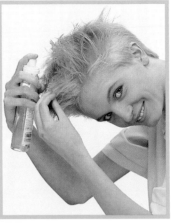 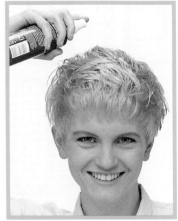

1 Start with hair that's clean and dry. Tip your head forwards and work volumising spray through to the roots.

2 Lift and mould the hair into shape with your fingers then lightly spritz with holding spray to fix in place.

SMART GIRLS KEEP IT SMOOTH

For a really sleek head of hair, use sprays to build in body and give a smooth finish.

Even sleek styles need movement, so hair mustn't be set like concrete. The secret is not to be too heavy-handed with spray – lightly does it!

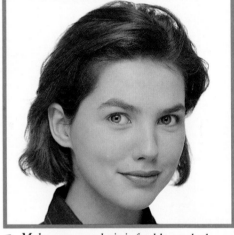

1 Make sure your hair is freshly-washed, towel-dried and free of tangles before you start to style it.

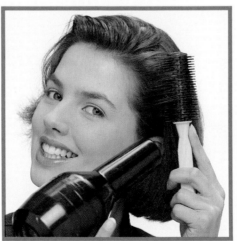

3 Blow-dry hair back off your face, using a round brush. Follow the brush with your hairdryer for a smooth finish.

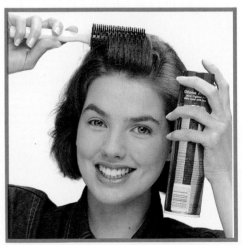

4 Now spritz with an aerosol hairspray, brushing it through from the roots to keep all hair smooth.

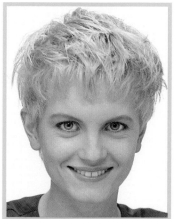

3 The finished result is a textured look that you can just fluff up again to revive.

LOOSEN UP

For a tousled look combine rough-drying with a volume spray.

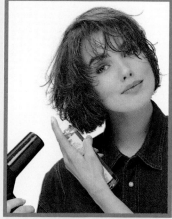

1 Start with towel-dried hair. Spritz with volumising spray, then tip your head to the side. Rough-dry with a hairdryer.

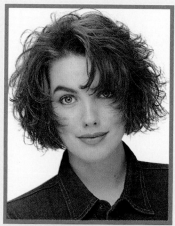

2 Dry all your hair in the same way, using your fingers to style and shape.

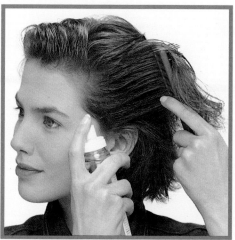

2 Run a vent brush through your hair, from roots to ends, at the same time spritzing with volumising spray.

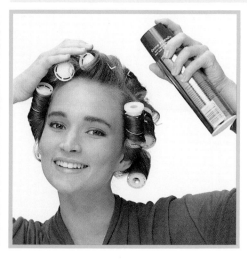

FINISHING TOUCHES

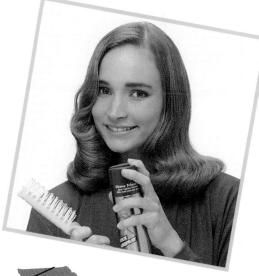

After setting your hair on heated rollers, lightly spritz with hairspray all over to help set the curls.

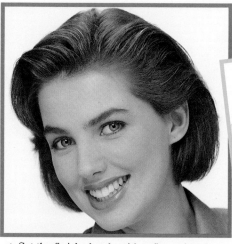

5 Set the finished style with a fine mist of hairspray all over. Smooth down any stray hairs with the palm of your hand.

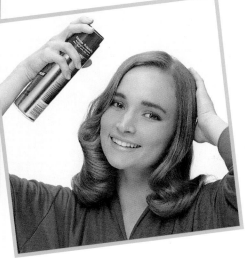

To give any style a less 'set' looking finish, squirt hairspray onto a brush, then run quickly through your hair before it dries.

Tip

Give a bob a sleek finish by spritzing hair lightly with hairspray then smoothing the hair under with your hand.

Photographs: ALISTAIR HUGHES/Hair: PENNY ATTWOOD/Make-up: DANIEL SANDLER/Denim shirt: TOP SHIRT/Brown blouse: HENNES/Lilac blouse: TOP SHOP/Taupe jacket: OASIS

STRAIGHT TO THE POINT

Smooth your fringe into pointed tips for a cheeky, impish look.

Salon secrets

For a really smooth finish, reverse your comb and use the back instead of the teeth.

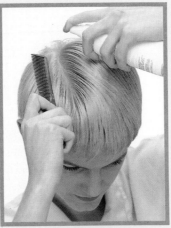

1 *Make a parting, if you wear one, then comb your hair smooth, following closely with a fine mist of styling spray.*

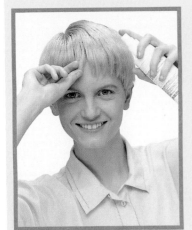

2 *Spritz the fringe with spray, teasing strands of hair into points with your fingers.*

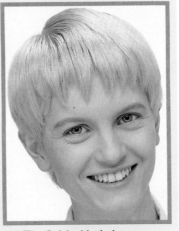

3 *The finished look draws attention to the eyes and flatters a fuller face.*

BACK TO YOUR ROOTS

Give lift to longer styles.

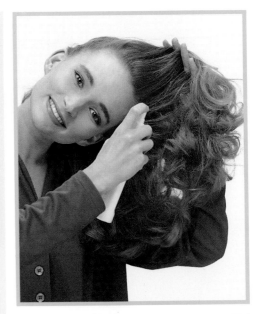

1 *Squirt holding spray directly at the hair between your fingers.*

2 *Tease out the curls at the ends of your hair, then use more spray to fix the style. Spray upwards so the style doesn't flop.*

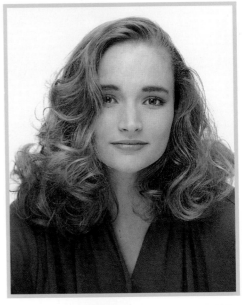

Watchpoint

If you have an elaborate style which needs a lot of spray to hold it, you may need to wash your hair more often to get rid of the build-up.

SCRUNCH IT UP

For a crisp, even curl on a layered bob, forget mousse and reach for the styling spray.

 Tip

Using spray rather than mousse to scrunch-dry fine, flyaway hair leaves it lots lighter.

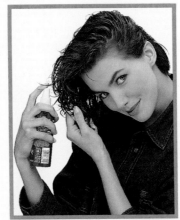

1 *Wash and towel-dry your hair, then tip your head forwards and squirt all over with styling spray, working it into the roots.*

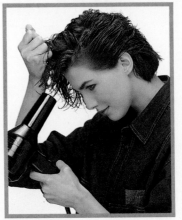

2 *Rough-dry all over with a hairdryer, then scrunch-dry by screwing up handfuls of hair and directing the dryer on to it.*

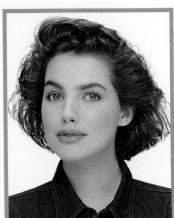

3 *The finished look shouldn't be too tight or too tousled. When it's just right, spritz with hairspray to hold.*

UPTOWN CURL

If your hair feels limp and lank then heat up your rollers and give yourself a headful of waves fit for a film star. You'll soon be ready to take on a starring rôle!

Photographs: ADRIAN BRADBURY/Hair: JENNI/Make-up: VIRGINIA NICHOLS/Coat: MONSOON.

BEFORE
Wash and dry your hair.

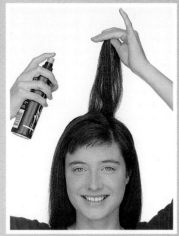

1 *Warm up your rollers then take a 5 cm/2 in wide section from the back of the crown, comb through and spray with hairspray.*

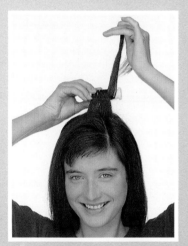

2 *Hold a roller about 5 cm/2 in above your head and wrap your hair around it to encourage more curl at the roots.*

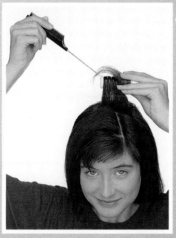

3 *Tuck any stray ends under the roller with the tail of a styling comb, and then secure with a roller pin.*

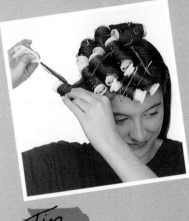

Tip

If you can't get the ends of your hair to stay put, wrap end papers around them before you fix the rollers to your head.

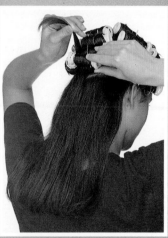

4 *Continue to wind rollers in horizontal sections down the back of your hair.*

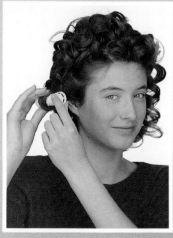

5 *When you've finished winding up the rollers, leave them in for 10 minutes before removing. Then leave the curls to cool.*

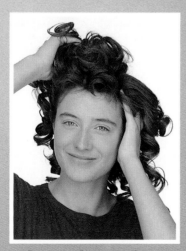

6 *Run your fingers gently through your hair to loosen the curls into waves.*

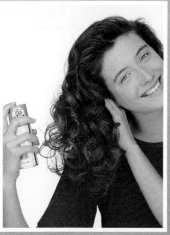

7 *Finish with a light spritz of spray-on shine. Be careful not to use too much or the curls will sag and hang flat.*

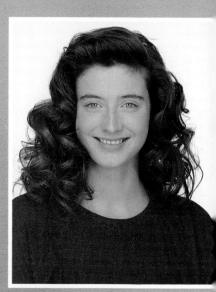

FINISHED

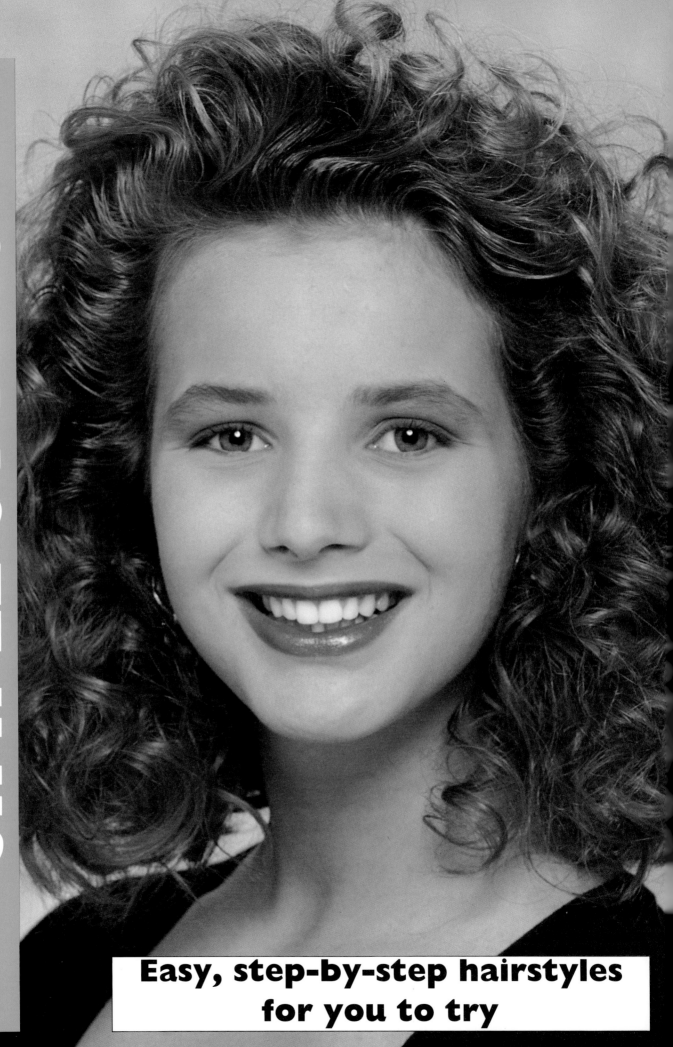

SIMPLE STYLES

Easy, step-by-step hairstyles for you to try

PERM HOLD!

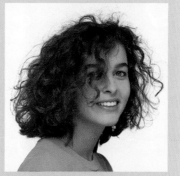

BEFORE
Start with dry hair, spritz with hairspray to give it extra hold.

Here's a topping idea for perking up your perm and livening up those layers

Personal styling guide

◆ *easy*

🕐 *quick to style*

✳ **Works best on** *permed or naturally curly hair that's chin-length or longer. Hair should be layered.*

☑ **You need:** *hairspray hairpins round brush*

FINISHED

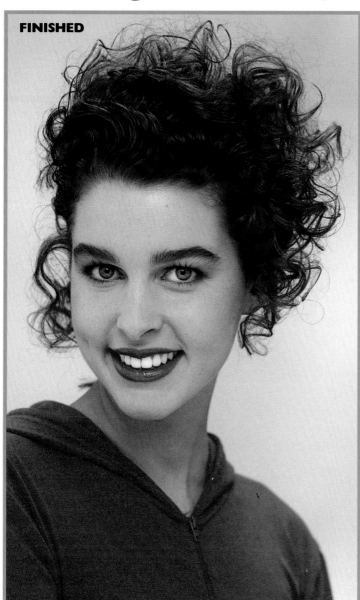

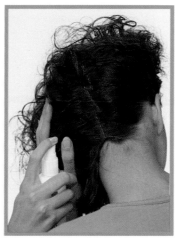

1 *Loosely take one side of your hair round to the back of your head and pin down the centre. Spritz with hairspray.*

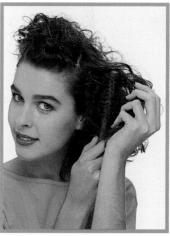

2 *Using a round brush, gently back-brush the front hair to add volume and height to the style.*

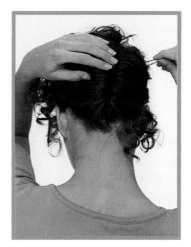

3 *Roll the length of your hair back to the centre and pin in place. Leave any stray ends loose.*

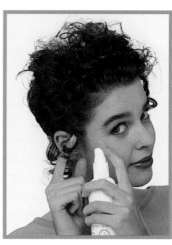

4 *Wind any loose tendrils around your finger and spritz with hairspray to hold the curl. The front should look tousled.*

Photographs: ALISTAIR HUGHES/Hair: JANE FOSTER/Make-up: VANESSA HAINES/Top: PINEAPPLE

FRENCH PLEAT

Pack a Parisian punch by updating a classic French pleat for a simple style that's the ultimate in continental chic

BEFORE
Start with clean dry hair.

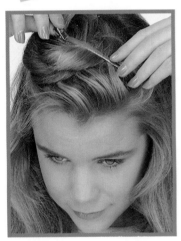

1 *Section off your hair at the front and clip out of the way – you'll work on this hair last.*

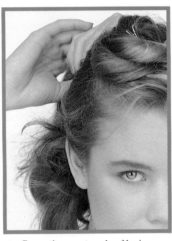

2 *Smooth on a touch of hair wax for sleekness and comb the rest of your hair into a ponytail at the back of your head.*

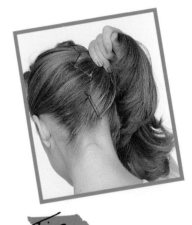

Tip
If your hair's fine, help the pleat to last by securing it with a line of criss-cross grips.

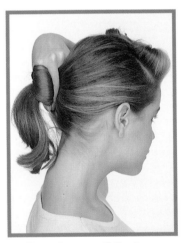

3 *Loop the ponytail firmly around your index finger and smooth with your comb.*

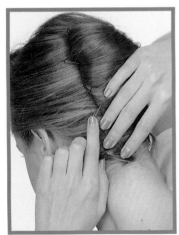

5 *Still holding firmly, twist your hand around until the hair on the outside of the roll is lying smooth. Secure with pins.*

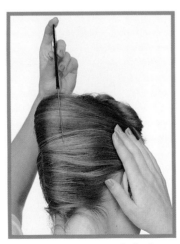

6 *Clean up any stray hairs by smoothing over with your tailcomb and hand.*

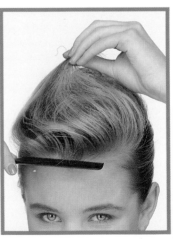

7 *Unpin the front section and back-comb lightly to add lift. Smooth back, keeping some wave in the hair.*

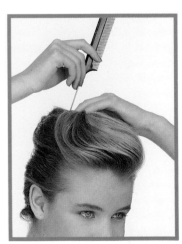

8 *Tuck the ends of your fringe into the top of the pleat with your tailcomb. Put a grip in and spritz with hairspray.*

Photographs: ADRIAN BRADBURY/Hair: LAURA for JOHN FRIEDA/Make-up: VIRGINIA NICHOLS/Top: MARY QUANT/Earrings: RIO

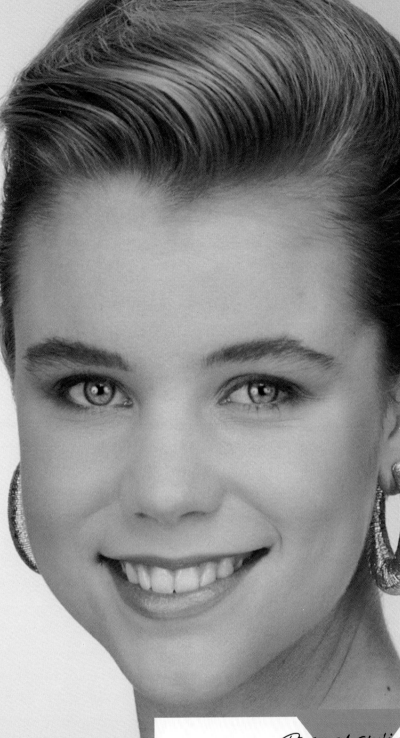

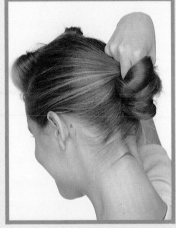

4 *Loop your hair around again until the ends are tucked in.*

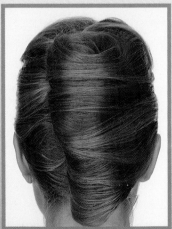

FINISHED

Personal styling guide

◆◆ some skill required

🕐 🕐 can't be hurried

✳ **Works best on** *straight or wavy shoulder-length hair.*

☑ **You need:**
tailcomb

hair grips
hair clips
styling wax
hairspray

~~Watchpoint~~

The pleat will look too bulky if your hair's long and thick.

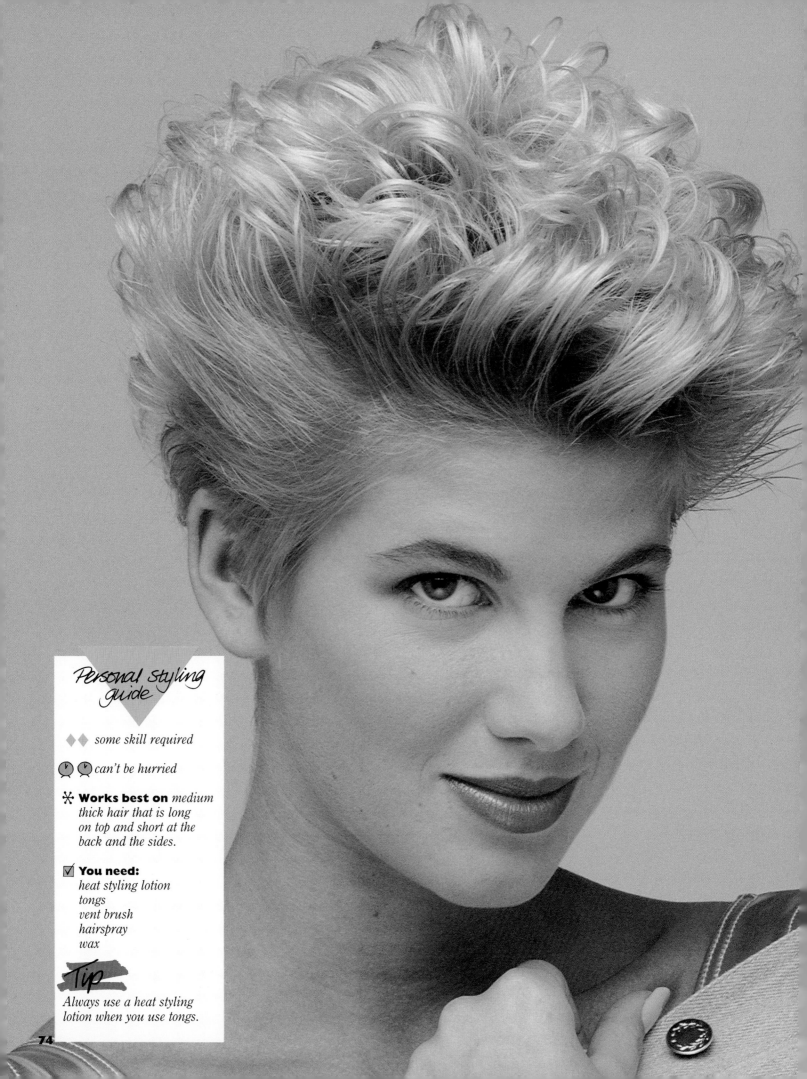

Personal styling guide

◆◆ *some skill required*

🕐🕐 *can't be hurried*

✳ **Works best on** *medium thick hair that is long on top and short at the back and the sides.*

☑ **You need:**
heat styling lotion
tongs
vent brush
hairspray
wax

Tip

Always use a heat styling lotion when you use tongs.

TONG-IN-CHIC

Give your hair a lift! Transform a smooth, long-layered style into masses of bubbly curls. It doesn't take long to master the technique — the secret lies in tonging the curls randomly

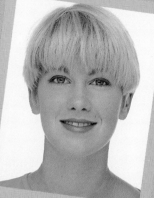

BEFORE
Make sure your hair is clean and completely dry before you begin to style it.

Photographs: PAUL MITCHELL/Hair: SHAUN GLOAG/
Make-up: LIZZIE COURT/Swimsuit: HENNES/Jacket: TOP SHOP

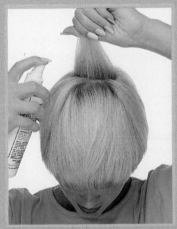

1 *Take a small section of hair from the back of your crown and spray lightly with heat styling lotion.*

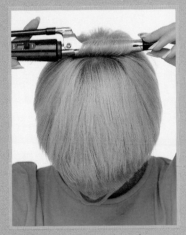

2 *Wrap the sprayed section around the heated styling tongs and hold in place for 30 seconds.*

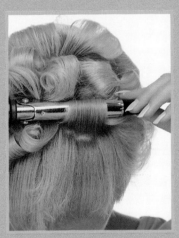

3 *Continue to make curls all over your head at random, positioning the curls so that there are no obvious partings.*

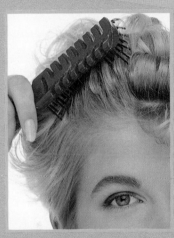

4 *Carefully brush the curls away from your face using a vent brush.*

FINISHED

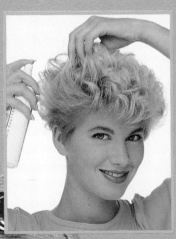

5 *Once you've arranged your hair just as you want it, fix the top in place with your usual hairspray.*

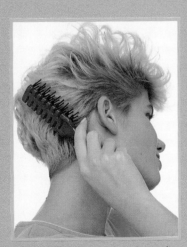

6 *Using your vent brush again, brush the sides of your hair backwards, sweeping it behind your ears.*

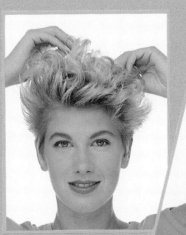

7 *Put a little hair wax on your fingertips and use it to break up your curls which will then take on a natural, shining look.*

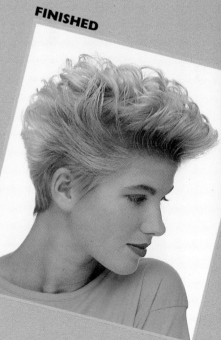

Photographs: PAUL MITCHELL/Hair: PENNY ATTWOOD/Make-up: KAREN LOCKYER/Dress: ZOO/Earrings: ACCESSORIZE

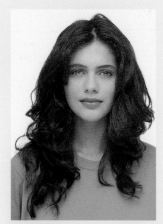

BEFORE
Don't shampoo for 24 hours before styling – natural oil will help.

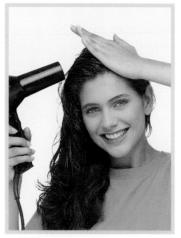

1 *Work a grapefruit-sized blob of mousse through the entire length of your hair. Dry the roots with your hairdryer.*

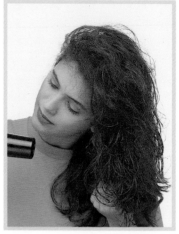

2 *Scrunch-dry the ends – lift the hair up in your fingers and scrunch it loosely to encourage the waves.*

TURN UP THE VOLUME

Long waves are where it's at! So get turned on to scrunch-drying and back-combing and make your stye a resounding success

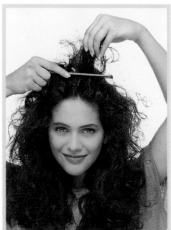

3 *Scrunch-dry top hair, then begin back-combing. Comb the hair around your face at the roots to create maximum body.*

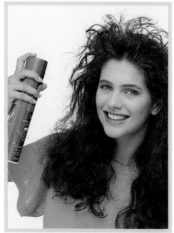

4 *Continue back-combing all the hair. Then spritz with plenty of hairspray at the roots to hold the back-combing in place.*

FINISHED
Hair has bags of body and great-looking waves.

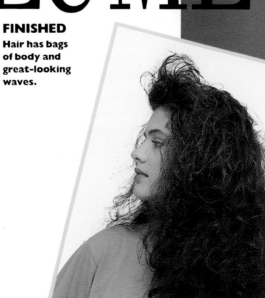

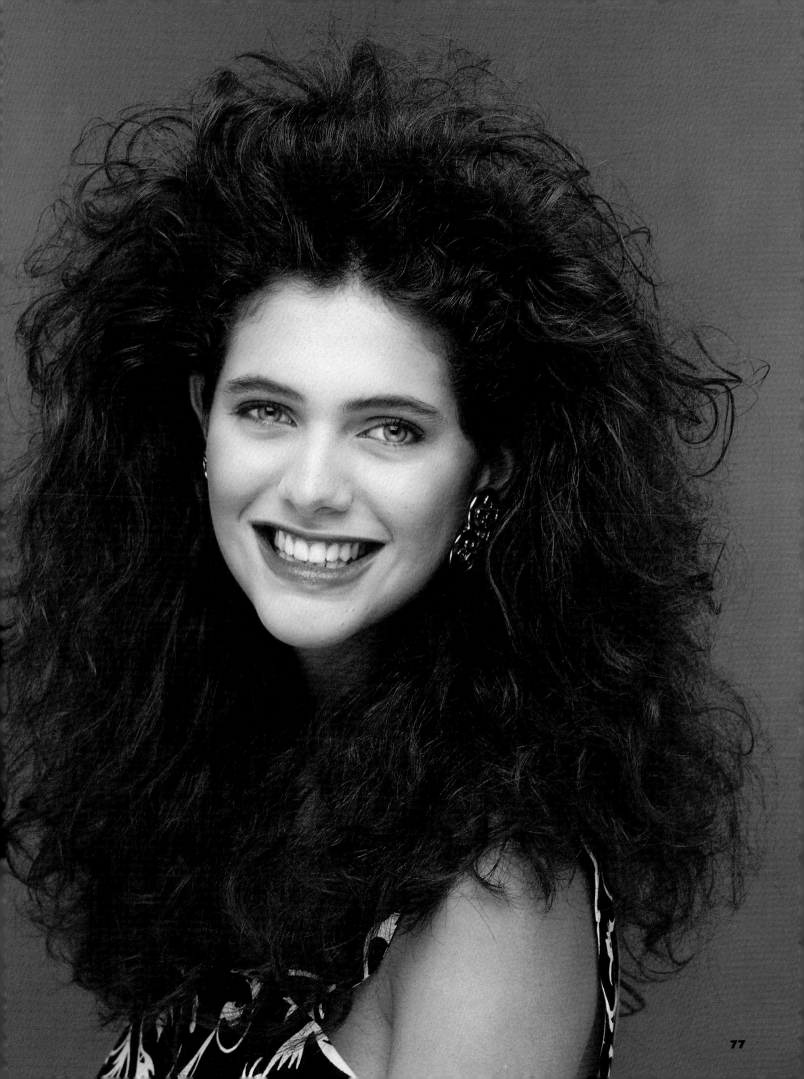

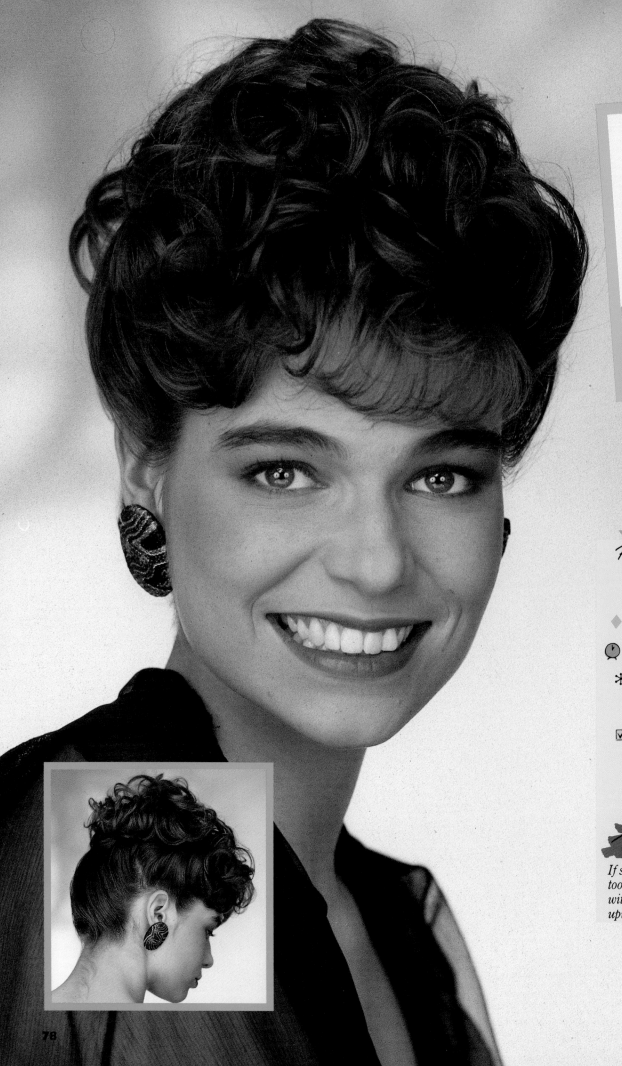

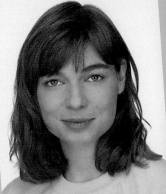

BEFORE
Make sure your hair is clean and dry before you start. Find your natural parting.

Personal styling guide

◆◆ some skill required

🕐🕐 can't be hurried

✳ **Works best on** shoulder length or longer hair.

☑ **You will need:**
heat styling lotion
hairdryer
curling tongs
hair grips
Afro comb

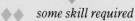

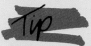

Tip

If some of your back hair is too short to gather up, spritz with hairspray and smooth it upwards to keep it in place.

78

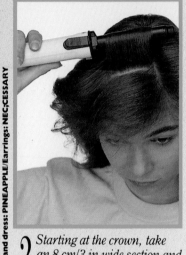

CURLS ON TOP

If your hair is neither long nor short but at that awkward in-between stage, don't let it get you down. Give yourself an instant lift with a topknot of tumbling curls

1 *Spray heat styling lotion through your hair. Set tongs to heat up. Rough-dry with a hairdryer for two minutes.*

Photographs: ADRIAN BRADBURY/Hair: JENNI/Make-up: VIRGINIA NICHOLS/Top and dress: PINEAPPLE/Earrings: NEC;CESSARY

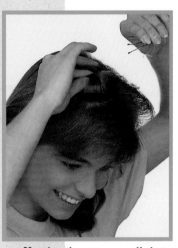

2 *Starting at the crown, take an 8 cm/3 in wide section and wind it onto the tongs. Hold for 30 seconds for a firm curl.*

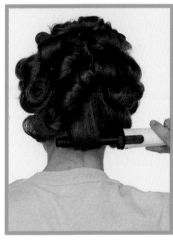

3 *Keeping the sausage-roll shape of the curl, secure it with a hair grip before starting to tong the rest of your hair.*

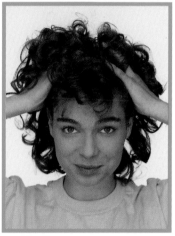

4 *Tong all over your hair so the curls lie in a random pattern, securing each curl as you go.*

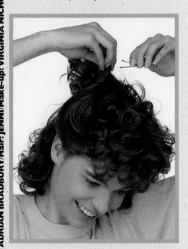

5 *Unclip the curls and gently work them loose with your fingers. Try not to pull them out of shape.*

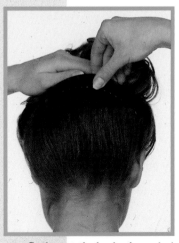

6 *Twist the side sections over once and gather up on top of your head. Secure with grips, leaving the curled ends free.*

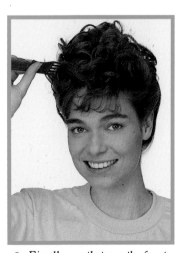

7 *Gather up the back of your hair in the same way, and use a wide, curved comb to give a smooth, secure finish.*

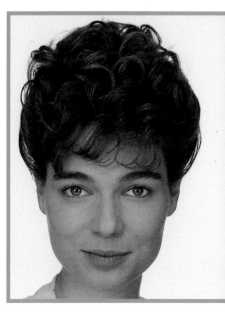

8 *Finally, gently tease the front curls with a wide-toothed comb to soften the fringe.*

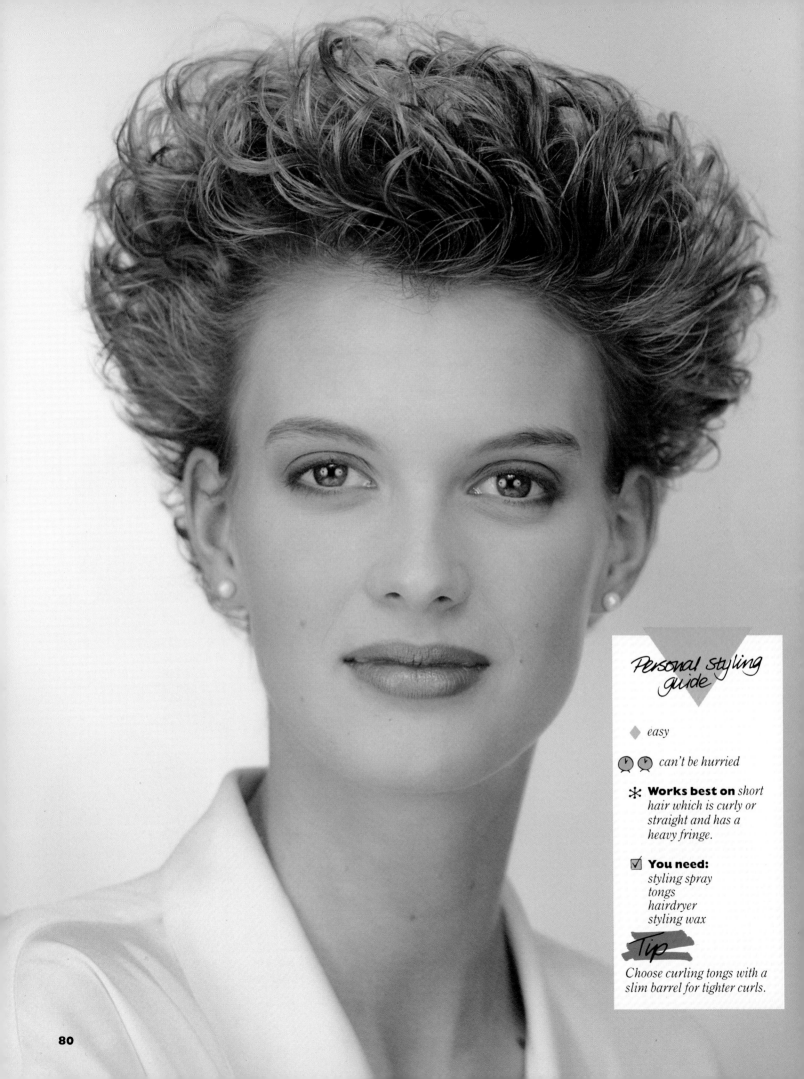

Personal styling guide

◆ *easy*

🕐🕐 *can't be hurried*

✳ **Works best on** *short hair which is curly or straight and has a heavy fringe.*

☑ **You need:**
styling spray
tongs
hairdryer
styling wax

Tip

Choose curling tongs with a slim barrel for tighter curls.

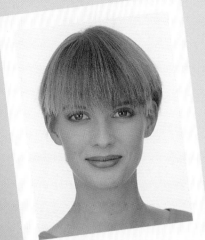

BEFORE
Comb through clean, dry hair to remove any knots and tangles. Spray lightly with styling spray.

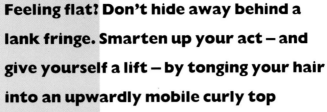

Feeling flat? Don't hide away behind a lank fringe. Smarten up your act – and give yourself a lift – by tonging your hair into an upwardly mobile curly top

STICK UP!

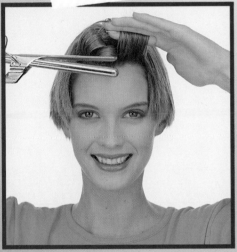

1 *Part your hair into 2.5 cm/1 in wide sections. Lift each vertically from your head and tong into sausage-shaped curls.*

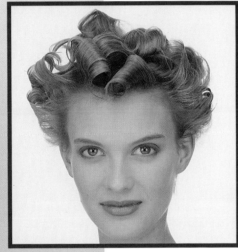

2 *Continue curling section by section until all the hair has been tonged into curls.*

For lasting hold on naturally straight or very fine hair finish off with a squirt of extra hold styling spray.

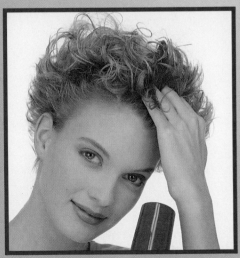

3 *Separate the curls by running your fingers vigorously through the hair, then tip your head forwards and blow-dry the roots.*

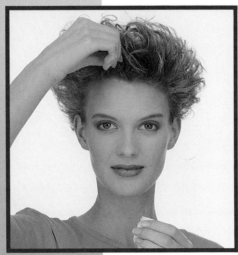

4 *A thumbnail-sized blob of styling wax worked through the hair will shape and separate the curls to finish the style.*

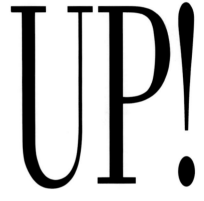

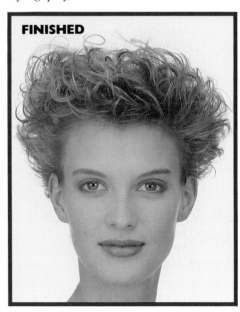

FINISHED

TWIST IN THE TAIL

Make some-fin more of your long hair with this elegant fishbone plait. Simply follow our guide and we're sure you'll soon be hooked on this look. So go on and splash out in style!

Photographs: ADRIAN BRADBURY/Hair: PENNY ATTWOOD/Make-up: SHARON IVES/Top: MISS SELFRIDGE/Earrings: CRYSTALIZE

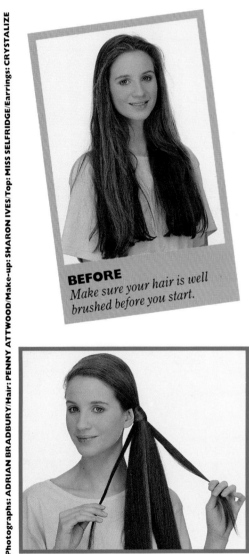

BEFORE
Make sure your hair is well brushed before you start.

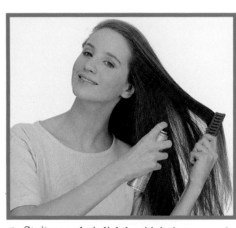

1 *Spritz your hair lightly with hairspray and brush it through thoroughly. This will help prevent static and give your plait a much neater finish.*

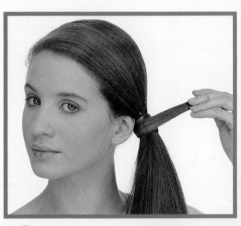

2 *Brush your hair over to one side then gather it into a ponytail, securing it with a covered elastic band. Take a strand of hair and wind it around the band, tuck in the end and secure with a hair grip.*

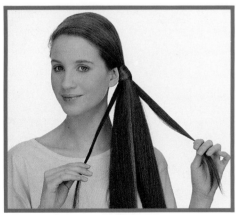

3 *Separate the ponytail into two bunches, then take a thin strand of hair from the outer section of each bunch.*

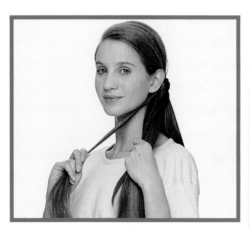

4 *Take the thin strand from the left-hand bunch over to the right and incorporate into the right-hand bunch.*

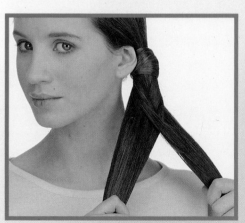

5 *Next take the thin strand from the right-hand bunch over to the left and incorporate into the left-hand bunch.*

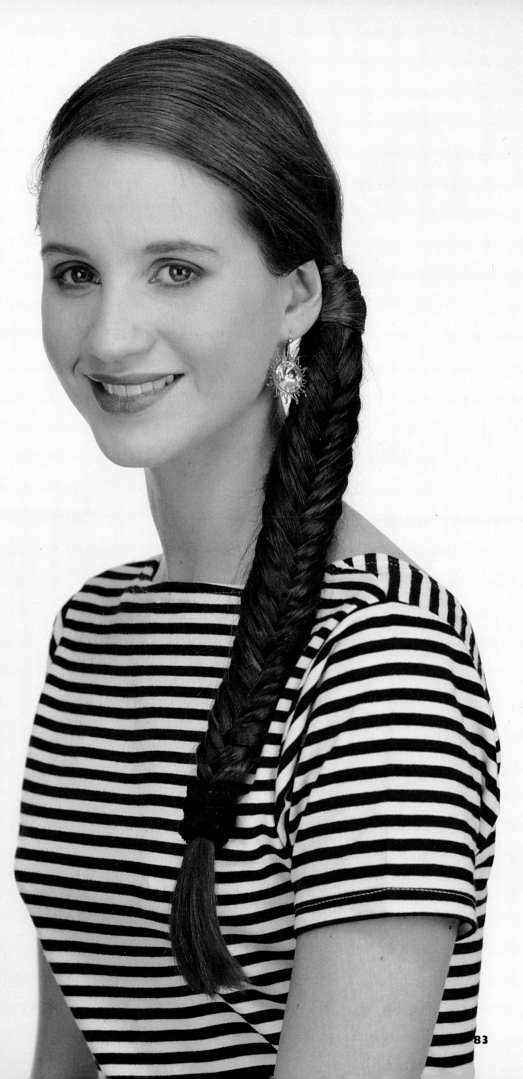

Personal styling
guide

◆◆   some skill required

🕐🕐   can't be hurried

✳ **Works best on** *hair*
that's all one length.

☑️ **You need:**
hairbrush
hairspray
covered elastic bands
hair grips

Tip

If your hair's curly or
wavy blow-dry it first for
a smooth finish.

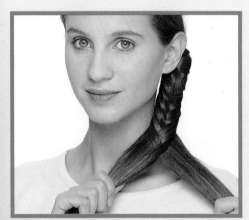

6 *Continue plaiting in this way down the length of hair taking in new strands as you work. Fasten the ends securely with a covered elastic band.*

CURLS AHEAD

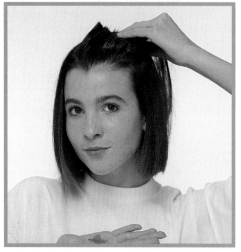

BEFORE
It's a sleek bob and in good condition, but sometimes it's nice to have a complete change.

Got a dead straight bob and thought you could do nothing with it? It might be sleek and smooth, but now's the time for a change. So get ahead, get a grip and get some curl!

1 *Switch on your tongs to heat up. Rub a marble-sized blob of gel through the length of your hair, being careful to distribute it evenly.*

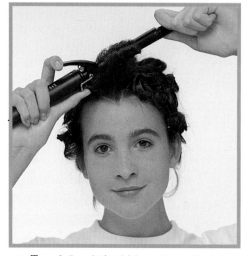

2 *Tong 2.5 cm/1 in-thick sections of hair into ringlets. Grip each ringlet to your head to help set the curl.*

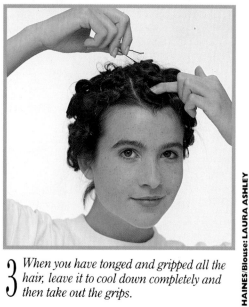

3 *When you have tonged and gripped all the hair, leave it to cool down completely and then take out the grips.*

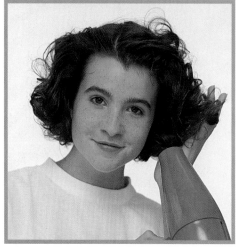

4 *Run your fingers through your hair to break the curl and, if it's still damp, scrunch-dry it with your hands and a hairdryer.*

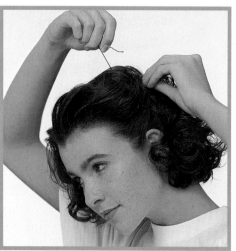

5 *Starting at one side, roll hair back behind your ear and loosely grip. Repeat on other side. Continue rolling up the rest of the hair.*

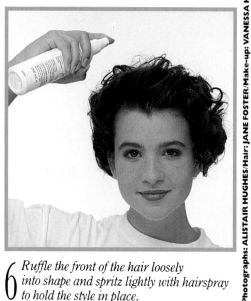

6 *Ruffle the front of the hair loosely into shape and spritz lightly with hairspray to hold the style in place.*

84

Photographs: ALISTAIR HUGHES/Hair: JANE FOSTER/Make-up: VANESSA HAINES/Blouse: LAURA ASHLEY

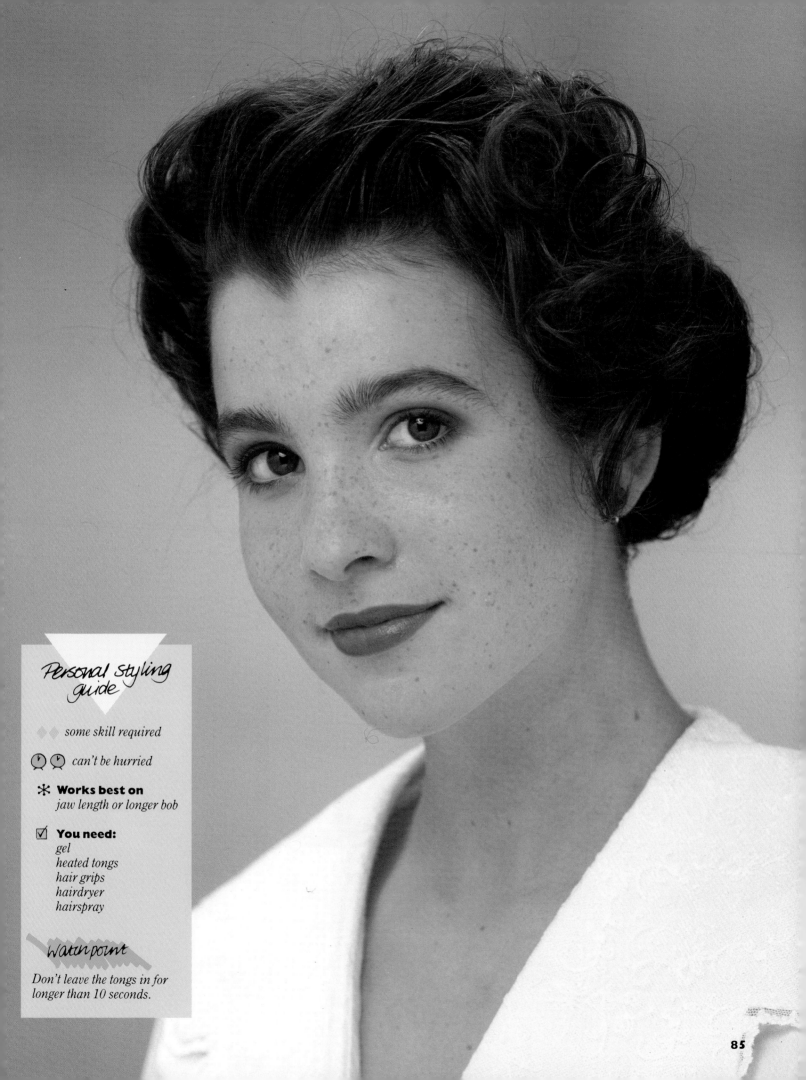

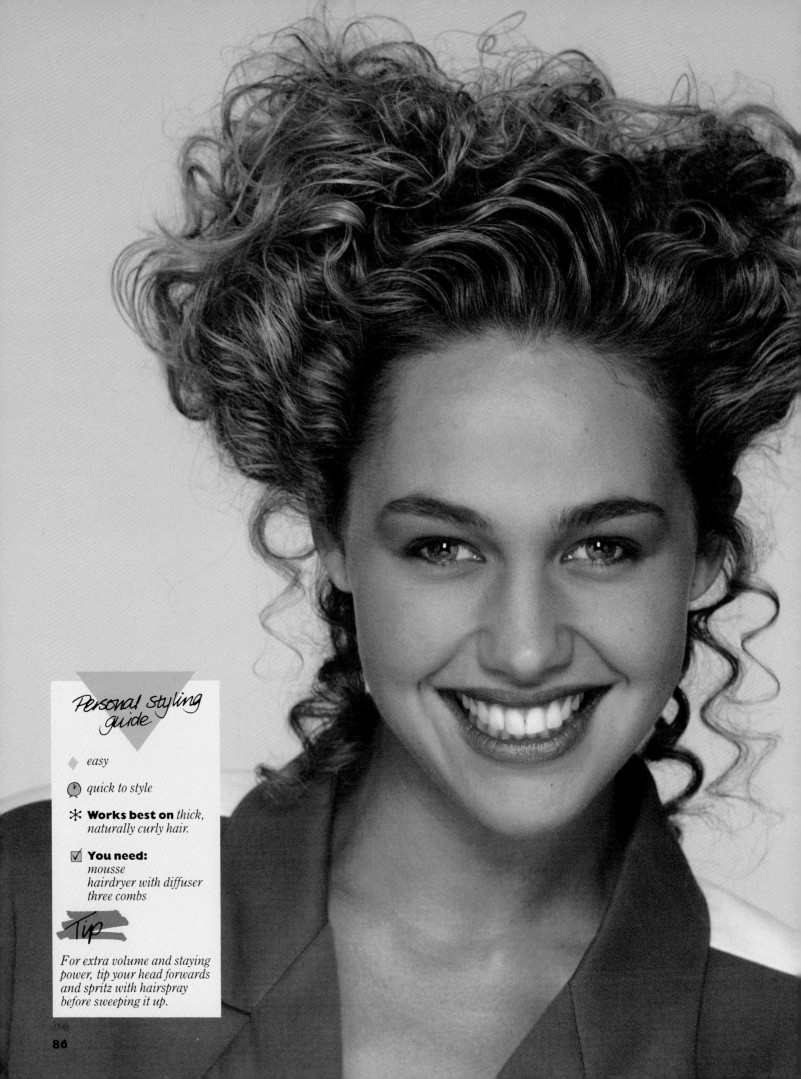

Personal styling guide

◆ *easy*

🕐 *quick to style*

✳ **Works best on** *thick, naturally curly hair.*

☑ **You need:**
mousse
hairdryer with diffuser
three combs

Tip

For extra volume and staying power, tip your head forwards and spritz with hairspray before sweeping it up.

PILE UP!

Go for the high life and tease wavy hair into luscious, tumbling curls. Quick and easy to style, it's worth a try if you're a girl who wants to be top of the pile!

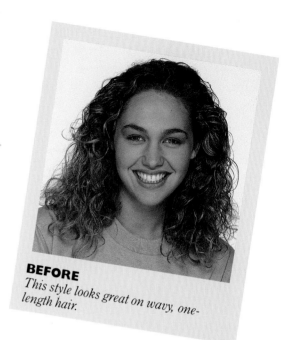

BEFORE
This style looks great on wavy, one-length hair.

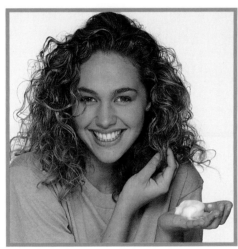

1 *Work through an egg-sized blob of mousse from roots to ends.*

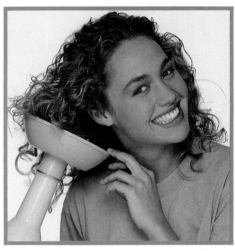

2 *Scrunch-dry your hair, attaching a diffuser to your hairdryer. For extra lift, tilt your head to the side.*

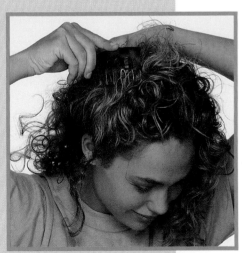

3 *Starting at one side, rake your hand through your hair taking it up towards the top of your head. Secure with a comb, letting any loose ends tumble over.*

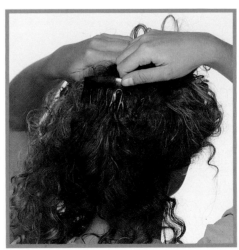

4 *Repeat at the back and other side of the head. Then gently ruffle and tease your hair into shape.*

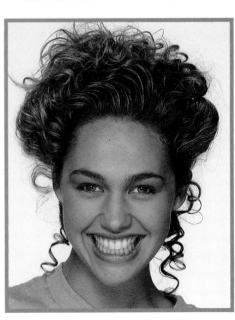

Photographs: NICK COLE/Make-up: KAREN PURVIS/Hair: JUSTIN/Jacket: NICK COLEMAN

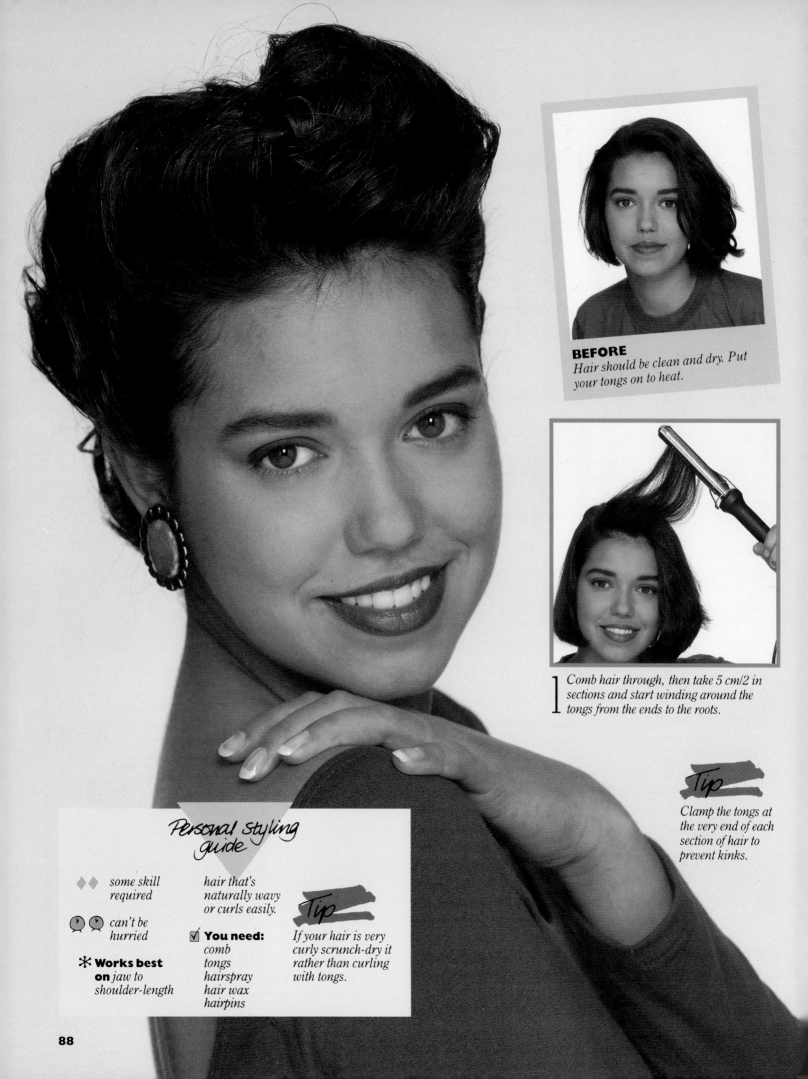

BEFORE
Hair should be clean and dry. Put your tongs on to heat.

1 *Comb hair through, then take 5 cm/2 in sections and start winding around the tongs from the ends to the roots.*

Tip

Clamp the tongs at the very end of each section of hair to prevent kinks.

Personal styling guide

♦♦ some skill required

🕐🕐 can't be hurried

✳ **Works best on** *jaw to shoulder-length*

hair that's naturally wavy or curls easily.

☑ **You need:**
comb
tongs
hairspray
hair wax
hairpins

Tip

If your hair is very curly scrunch-dry it rather than curling with tongs.

UP AND OVER

A classic bob looks lovely left loose, but if you want to be more daring try tonging in curls — then rolling them off your face for a really fabulous finish!

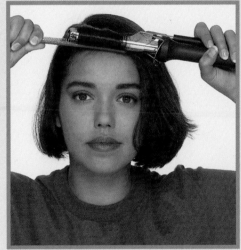

2 *As you wind, place a comb through each section so that it lies flat against the scalp to protect it from the heat. Hold for 30 seconds.*

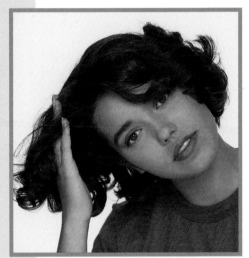

3 *When you have tonged all your hair, gently ruffle your hair with your fingers to break up the curl and give added volume.*

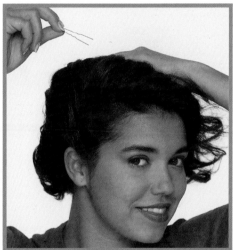

4 *Gather up one side of your hair and roll back and tuck. Use hairpins to secure the roll in place. Repeat on the other side.*

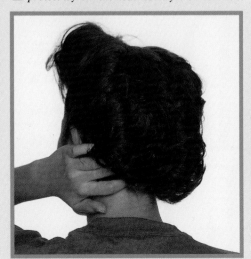

5 *When you have rolled both sides finish the back of the hair by running your fingers through to fan the hair out.*

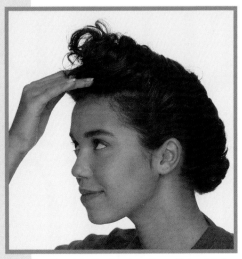

6 *Finally, style the front section. For added shine, rub a little wax on your fingertips and run them through your hair.*

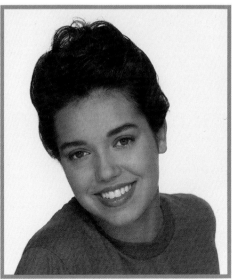

FINISHED

Photographs: NICK COLE/Hair: PENNY ATTWOOD/Make-up: LIZZIE COURT/Top: PINEAPPLE/Earrings: HENNES

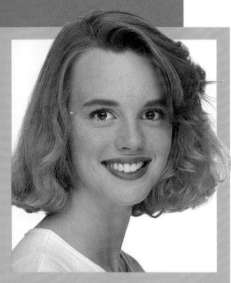

BEFORE
Hair is slightly wavy at the ends.

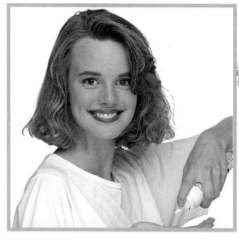

1 *Put the tongs on to heat up. Massage an orange-sized blob of mousse through slightly damp hair – working from the roots to the ends.*

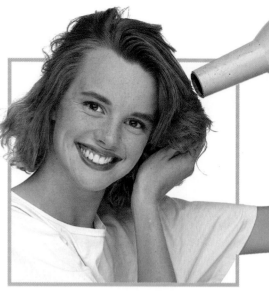

2 *Rough-dry your hair with a hairdryer. Make sure it's completely dry all over before you start tonging.*

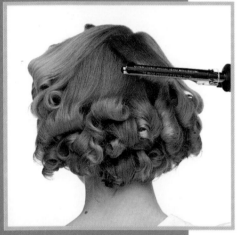

3 *Taking 2.5 cm/1 in sections, tong the underneath nape hair first, then work up towards the crown. Hold each curl for around 10 seconds.*

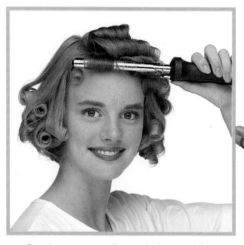

4 *Continue to tong all your hair – working round to the front until you have masses of sausage-shaped curls.*

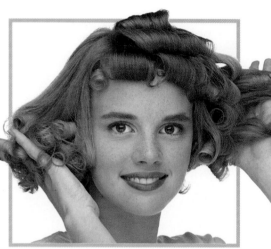

5 *Break the curls up into gentle waves by running your fingers through them. Don't brush your hair – you'll pull the curl out.*

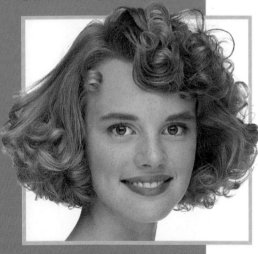

6 *The finished look – the full curls hide a frizzy, growing-out perm. Spritz with hairspray to hold the curls in place.*

SHARP TONGED!

With a flick of the tongs you can transform a wilting perm into perfect curls

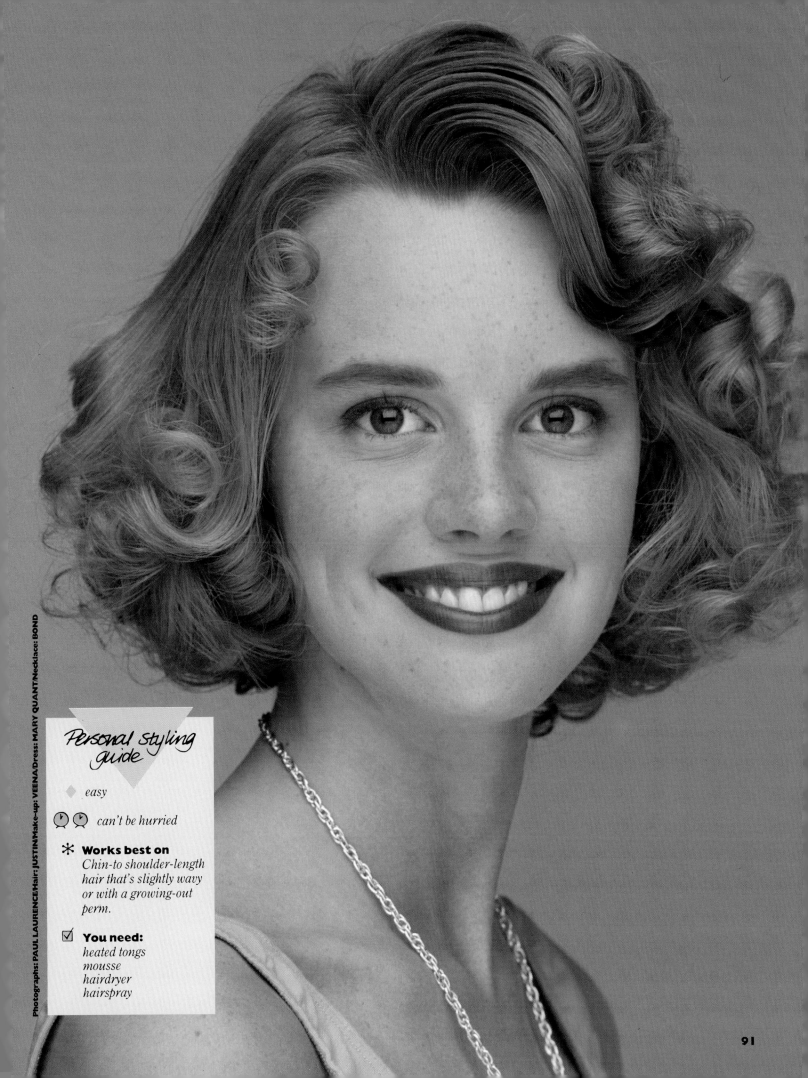

Personal styling guide

◆ *easy*

🕐🕐 *can't be hurried*

✳ **Works best on**
Chin-to shoulder-length hair that's slightly wavy or with a growing-out perm.

☑ **You need:**
heated tongs
mousse
hairdryer
hairspray

91

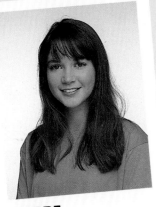

BEFORE
Clean roots are essential because they're going to be on display. Brush your hair thoroughly first.

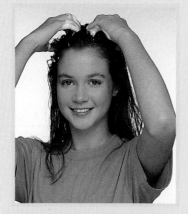

1 *Dampen hair all over with a water spray, then work an orange-sized blob of mousse through from the roots to the ends.*

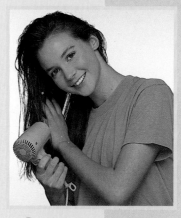

2 *Rough dry hair using a hot setting on your dryer to create texture and body.*

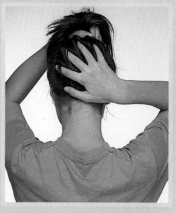

3 *Use your fingers to sweep your hair up into a ponytail on your crown. Fasten with a covered elastic band.*

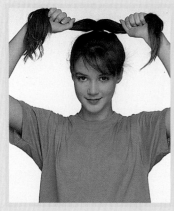

4 *Divide the ponytail into two equal sections and gently tug to make sure the root hair is pulled tight.*

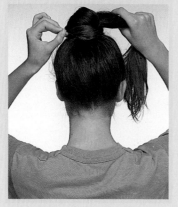

5 *Wind one section over and around the base of the other section. Tuck ends under at the back and hold with hairpins.*

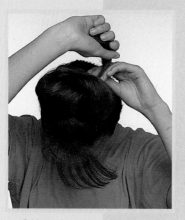

6 *Lift the second section so that it crosses over the back of the first one. Loop hair round then tuck ends under neatly. Use hairpins to hold hair in place.*

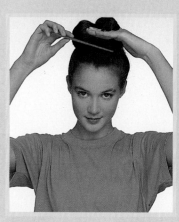

7 *Back-comb the roots of your fringe, then comb it over to one side so that it forms a quiff.*

DOUBLE CROSSER!

Feel you need to smarten up your act a little? Step into the spotlight with this glamorous, upswept style and give long hair a dual role

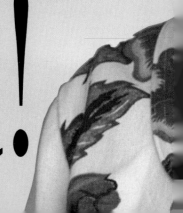

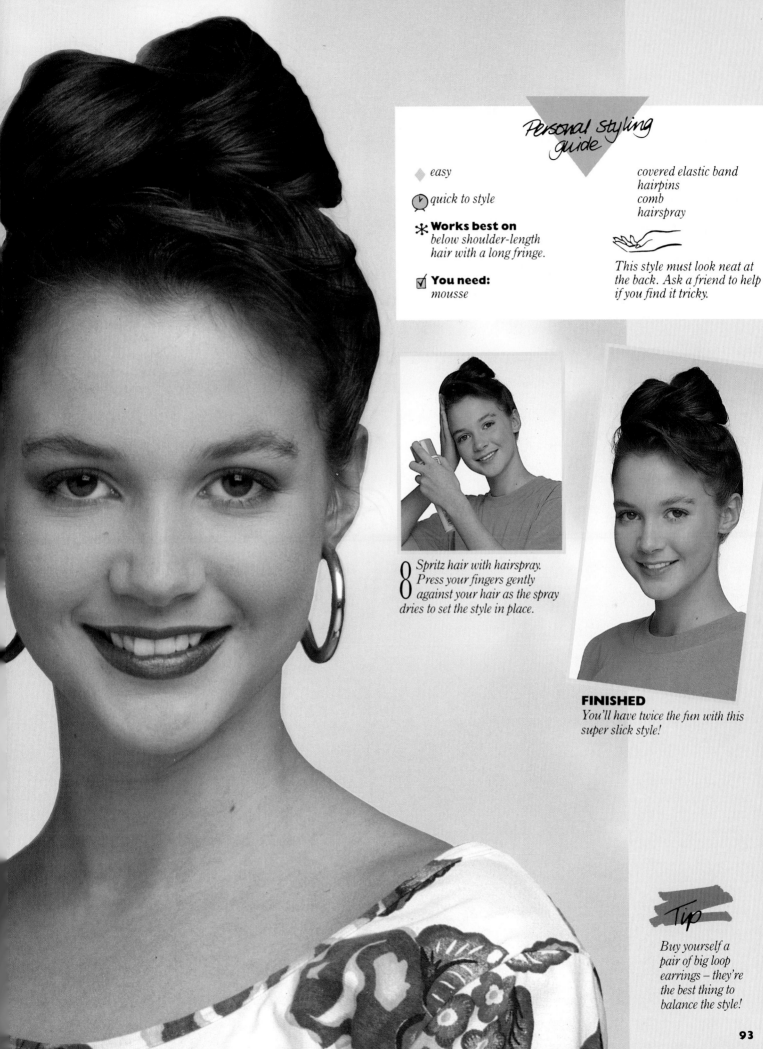

◆ easy

🕐 quick to style

✳ **Works best on**
below shoulder-length
hair with a long fringe.

☑ **You need:**
mousse

covered elastic band
hairpins
comb
hairspray

This style must look neat at
the back. Ask a friend to help
if you find it tricky.

8 Spritz hair with hairspray.
Press your fingers gently
against your hair as the spray
dries to set the style in place.

FINISHED
You'll have twice the fun with this
super slick style!

Tip

Buy yourself a
pair of big loop
earrings – they're
the best thing to
balance the style!

Photographs: MATTHEW SMITH/Hair: PENNY ATTWOOD/Make-up: KAREN PURVIS/Top: FRENCH CONNECTION

TOP LOOK

Two in one — a body-building style that's worth its weight in gold. Plus a slicker version that's only a brush-stroke away. With either one you're hall-marked for success!

Personal styling guide

◆ *easy*

◷ *quick to style*

✳ **Works best on** *medium to thick, one-length hair.*

☑ **You need:**
*mousse
diffuser
hairdryer
comb
hairspray
brush*

Photographs: ALISTAIR HUGHES/Make-up: NICOLA ROSS/Hair: PAULA MANN/Tops: MARY QUANT, WAREHOUSE
Blouse: WAREHOUSE/Earrings: ACCESSORIZE, TRIFARI

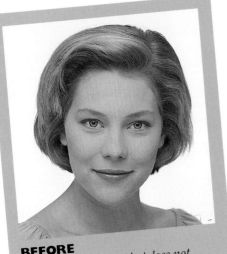

BEFORE
Hair should be clean but does not need to be newly-washed.

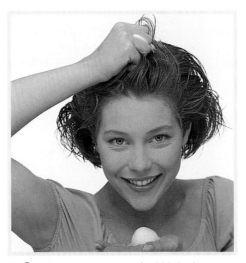

1 *Squeeze out an orange-sized blob of mousse and work it right through your hair so all the strands are evenly covered.*

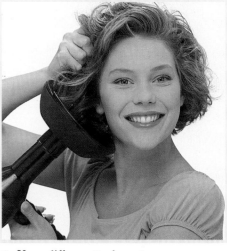

2 *Use a diffuser attachment on your hairdryer and scrunch-dry. Direct the air jet from below to create width.*

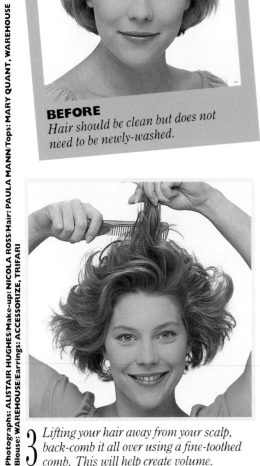

3 *Lifting your hair away from your scalp, back-comb it all over using a fine-toothed comb. This will help create volume.*

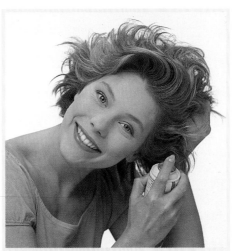

4 *Spritz the roots of your hair with your favourite hairspray. Drop your head forward to get fullness at the back.*

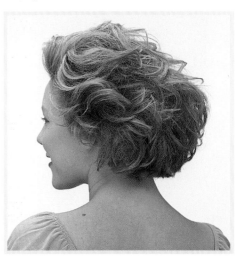

5 *Use your fingers to position your hair away from your face for a fabulous backswept look. Spritz with hairspray again.*

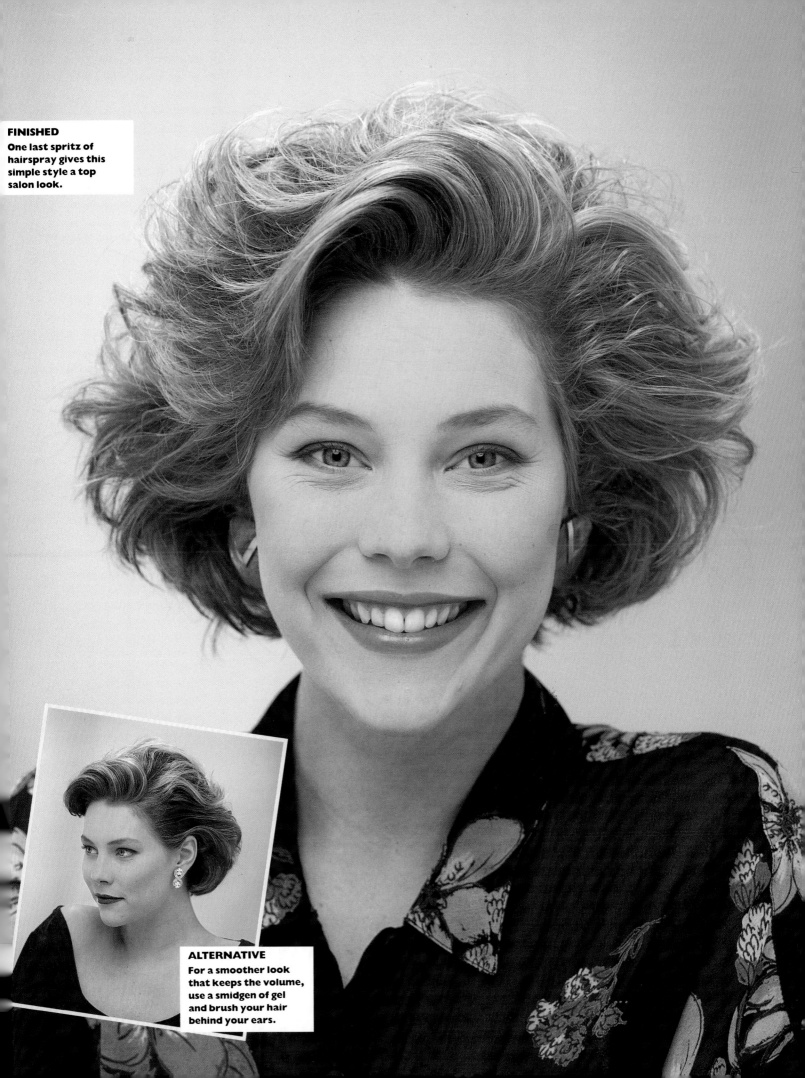

FINISHED
One last spritz of hairspray gives this simple style a top salon look.

ALTERNATIVE
For a smoother look that keeps the volume, use a smidgen of gel and brush your hair behind your ears.

INDEX